Faith
Through the
Feminine

A Biblical Approach to Menstruation,
Cycle Syncing, and All Things Women's Health

Alycia Hammer

HU
HOUSE
PUBLISHING

HEARTS UNLEASHED HOUSE PUBLISHING

Copyright © 2025 Hearts Unleashed House Publishing

Text copyright © 2025 by Alycia Hammer
Cover design © 2025 by Alycia Hammer
Interior book layout by Susan Harring © 2025 by Alycia Hammer

For information about special discounts for bulk purchases contact:
abigail@heartsunleashed.com

Manufactured in the United States of America
Library of Congress Cataloging-in-Publication Data Hammer, Alycia.

Summary:

Faith Through the Feminine explores the deep and often overlooked connections between biblical faith and women's health, specifically menstruation and the menstrual cycle.

In this book, Hammer challenges the idea that the Bible is male-centric by encouraging readers to look for and embrace the feminine aspects of Scripture.

Through personal stories, biblical analysis, and health coaching insights, this book reframes menstruation as a God-designed process worthy of respect and reverence.

ISBN: 978-1-968201-04-3

[1. Christian Women's Health. 2. Biblical Womanhood. 3. Menstrual Health & Spirituality. 4. Faith and Wellness. 5. Women in the Bible. 6. Religious Self-Help for Women. 7. Feminine Spirituality.]

To the women of God who were never told that their bodies
and all their functions were sacred and mirrored in the Bible.
This book is my prayer for your healing, your confidence,
and deepening your relationship with Jesus.

Acknowledgments

First and foremost, this book was only made possible because of God's guidance. Every time I was stuck in my writing, He led me back to His word and reminded me of the focus of my book.

A huge thank you to my husband and children for giving me the time and space to research, write, and pray over this book. God has blessed me with the most supportive family and friends.

Table of Contents

Part 1

Focus on the Feminine

When you think about the Bible, what comes to mind? Femininity? Menstruation? Women's health? Many women have been told the lie that the Bible is male-centric; written by men, for men, about men. They believe that women are just the side story and supporting characters. If you were told your whole life that the Bible isn't for women or about women, you might read the Bible noticing that it isn't for you. What if you read the Bible with the focus on femininity? When you are actively looking for femininity in the Bible, you will start seeing more and more of it. Focus on the feminine.

Early in my writing journey, I shared the vision for my book with a friend who lovingly commented, "Wow! How did you come up with that idea? It almost sounds like a college thesis taking two unrelated things and showing how they're connected." And that's exactly it. We are God's children created in His image. The Bible is His story of creation and life. Femininity and the Bible are not unrelated at all. The Bible is just as much for women as it is for men.

Have you ever thought of your womanly cycle as a biblical experience? If not, you're not alone. Becoming a woman is a monumental milestone in your life marked by the coming of your first period. It's your body's way of saying you are ready, physically, to conceive children and it's a monthly check-in for your overall health. This time of your life is a great time of transformation and renewal. Some navigate it with the grace of a swan and others handle it like a bull in a china shop.

The day I became a woman is a day I will never forget. My twelfth Christmas came the same way it always did—exciting and busy. I was blissfully unaware that one of my favorite holidays was about to turn bloody. When I went to the bathroom at my aunt's house, taking a much needed introvert break from my large family gathering, I looked down and saw them—the red drops of womanhood.

At first I doubted what I saw. This couldn't possibly be my period; I was just seeing things. Then reality started to sink in and along with it came the panic. *I'm not at home! I'm not prepared for this! What should I do?* I wasn't able to yell across the family party to get my mom to help me. And what would everyone say if they found out? I was stuck in a spiral of embarrassment and sadness. This wasn't how it was supposed to happen. I'd spent the last couple years eager to become a woman—at home in the comfort of my bathroom stocked with all the proper feminine hygiene products. I had this idea that my mom would bring me a warm water bottle or heating pad to put on my abdomen and we would relax on the couch watching girly movies while eating our favorite snacks. This was far from my perfect image of how this was all going to go down.

Deep in the dark shadows of my brain hid the information I learned in fourth grade during "the talk," but we never covered "ruining your Christmas with your period" in any of the segments. I calmed myself down, stuffed some toilet paper in my underwear and suffered the rest of the evening with embarrassment wadded up in my pants.

Not only did I feel this ruined Christmas for me, to top it all off, the one friend I told in secret about my plunge into womanhood let the cat out of the bag to other people at school. I wanted to crawl into a hole and never come out. (Exaggeration was my love language at the time.) The embarrassment over my body, the shame and grossness I felt about myself, were crushing me. My life felt like it was over.

To my surprise, life continued on. No one actually cared that I got my period (even though I felt like everyone cared, gossiped about it, and thought about it all the time…because…I was twelve). Every girl at school eventually got their own period at one point in the next few years and it became more taboo to not have your period than to have it. However, it was still a topic that was more often than not met with groans and negative feelings like shame, embarrassment, and ick. To this day, aside from a woman relieved to have her period due to an unplanned pregnancy scare, the common reaction to "that time of the month" is, "Ugh." It's not typically excitement, it's not gratefulness. It's seen as an undesirable necessity, an inconvenience, of life as a woman.

Becoming a woman is a deeply personal and spiritual event in every woman's life. Think back to your first period. Perhaps your very first period is a blur and the details are foggy or maybe you have a vivid memory of where you were, how you felt, what you were wearing, the smell in the air, and how you perceived others' reactions to your period. Maybe you celebrated becoming a woman, maybe your womanhood was met with dread, or maybe it was somewhere in between.

I remember my first period because I had a lot of emotions around the big day. I was so excited to get my period until it actually showed up. Not everyone has an emotionally charged story to share about their first period and I know that not everyone feels the same way about their menstruation. I have found, though, that many women share common negative themes about the natural functions of their bodies: shame, embarrassment, and disgust. This is not a blanket statement for all women, however, it is, sadly, not uncommon for a woman to experience some sort of negative body image in her life—be it around her period or other parts of her body. I have been able to shed my negative feelings toward my period and my body after digging into my faith through femininity, and I hope this book will free you of any of those negative body images as well.

When I tell people I'm writing a book, their first question, naturally, is, "What is your book about?" I very confidently share that my book is about how menstruation and women's health are intimately tied to the Bible. I give a quick synopsis about what my book is about and watch for their reaction. My topic has been met with equal parts awkwardness and excitement. It's time we ditch the awkward and focus on the excitement.

I was born and raised in the Catholic Church. While I haven't always been close to the Church, I've always been close to my faith and when I started to explore the Bible more, I started to see a lot of connections from scripture to women's health; specifically the menstrual cycle. I've found a lot of comfort and have been able to shed a lot of shame through the Bible. Don't geat me wrong, I don't offer up the information about having my period to every person I see, but when the topic does come up, I don't squirm and feel awkward like I used to. I can confidently speak about having my period sans shame. My hope for you is that you will be able to see your body as the most precious and amazing creation by God and can shed your shame or any negativity you have through Jesus.

My interpretations of what the Bible is saying may be different than your interpretations. And that is okay. Everyone has their own world view impacting the way interpretations are made. While reading the Bible and thinking about these connections, I did my due diligence to explore alternative views and really think about what God is telling us. While I'm not a theologian, I am a certified Integrative Nutrition Health Coach specialized in hormones. My mission is to support women in their health journeys through trusting God's creation.

Before I started to think about my cycle in a faith-based way, I dreaded my period. Now that I see my faith through my body— my temple—I actually love having it. It's a reminder that Jesus bled on the cross to give us life just as a woman has to bleed in order to be able to give life to the world. Your first period was the beginning of womanhood and your body announcing you can now conceive. That is so huge! It's something that calls for a celebration, but is so often met with embarrassment, shame, fear, disgust, confusion, and all around negativity.

This book was not only written to explain and enhance your

understanding of how your faith affects how you view your periods, but also to explain how you can support your body through each phase of your cycle and overall health in a faith-based way. It's quite amazing how much of our cycles are mirrored in the stories of the Bible and I hope you will not only feel a sense of acceptance and lose any sense of shame or embarrassment around the topic, but also see how your body's cycles can be a religious experience. It is something to be celebrated and honored instead of shamed and silenced. I'm not suggesting you take to the streets and shout out that you have your period, but rather to be open about it with yourself and those who love and support you. If you are a man reading this; maybe to support your wife or just get a better understanding of women, I applaud you. This is, of course, fundamentally written for women to better support and accept their God-given bodies, but serious kudos to the men in our lives who want to know more.

Jesus Loves You for Who You Are

While certain parts of the Bible can evoke negative feelings of having a period, stories in the New Testament promote Jesus' love for all of us—including menstruating women. In Matthew we see a story about how Jesus reacted to a woman who was bleeding and in this one story alone, I find great solace.

To give some context to this part of Matthew's story, Jesus was on his way to a synagogue leader's home to heal the man's twelve-year-old daughter. The girl had already died, and Jesus was about to raise her from the dead. On his way to the man's daughter, he was approached from behind by a woman. The rest of Matthew 9:20-22 (NIV) goes like this: "Just then a woman who had been subject to bleeding for twelve years came up behind him [Jesus] and touched the edge of his cloak. She said to herself, 'If I only touch his cloak, I will be healed.' Jesus turned and saw her. 'Take heart, daughter,' he said, 'your faith has healed you.' And the woman was healed at that moment."

This is a monumental event that can often be overlooked. But before I'm able to fully express how huge this simple touch was at the time, it's important to take a look at the Old Testament. Leviticus 15:19-23 (NIV) says, "When a woman has her regular flow of blood, the impurity of her monthly period will last seven days, and anyone who touches her will be unclean till evening. Anything she lies on during her period will be unclean, and anything she sits on will be unclean. Anyone who touches anything she sits on will be unclean; they must wash their clothes and bathe with water, and they will be unclean till evening."

According to Leviticus, women are unclean and impure and anyone who touches a menstruating woman is also unclean and impure for the rest of the day. Jesus did not lash out at the woman for touching Him and making Him impure and unclean. He didn't reject her or hold any resentment for her actions. No. He calls her daughter and treats her with love then moves on to raise a little girl from the dead. He didn't stop and turn around because He had been touched by an unclean woman. The woman healed from bleeding had faith in Jesus and that alone made her well. What a powerful story for women!

When reading the Bible, it is very easy to feel like God had it out for women or that the Bible is all for men—especially when you read Leviticus in the Old Testament. The Leviticus verse about women being unclean and impure stopped me in my tracks the first time I read it. I'm unclean and impure for having my period?! It's not my fault this happens, I didn't choose to get my period. Deep frustration began to brew inside of me. I thought *if this isn't proof that this was written by a man, I don't know what is.* But before I let my frustration take over me, I kept reading and realized God wasn't keen on men's discharge either as shown in Leviticus:

Leviticus 15:16 (NIV) "When a man has an emission of semen, he must bathe his whole body in water and be unclean till evening."

While this made me feel less like the Bible had it out for my natural bodily functions, I digress back to the main point: Leviticus in the Old Testament does not come off as friendly to menstruation.

As I started to dig into my interpretation of these verses in the Bible and their use of the words "unclean" and "impure" I came up with a literal interpretation and one that required me to think as a historian; meaning I needed to think from the lens of the people and their beliefs at the time it was written. So literally would be that yes, indeed, our periods are unclean. These women during the time of the Bible were not using their menstrual cups, discs, tampons, or even nice absorbent pads. They had extra fabric—if they were lucky—to keep between their legs. So yes. It was a messy, unclean time for women—literally.

Then I thought about the idea of "unclean" and "impure" as a historian. Just because something is unclean or impure, it does not mean it is sinful. Whew! That's a relief. It's easy to read those words and feel shame in not wanting to be sinful or "bad," but have no fear! This does not mean you are being sinful or are forgotten or punished by God in any way.

Don't just take my word for it, though. Let's look at the Bible to see what it says. Have you heard the story of Noah and his awesome ark? God instructed Noah to build an ark large enough for his family and two of every animal—clean <u>and unclean</u>. Everyone ridiculed Noah for building a giant boat in the middle of a desert, but Noah followed God's calling anyway. When the rains came and flooded the lands, Noah's family and the animals brought aboard had the honored task of repopulating the world. If God didn't love or desire the unclean animals, He would not have instructed Noah to take them with him on the ark. He could have rid the world of the unclean animals in the flood, but He didn't because being unclean does NOT mean unloved or sinful or unworthy in the eyes of God.

During the time that Leviticus was written, a woman was praised and valued for her abilities to procreate, which she was not doing when menstruating. Therefore women would be seen as impure because the goal of the time was to populate the world to spread the faith. Men are also said to be unclean in the Bible for their discharge which, again, wouldn't bring about children. In order to spread the faith, believers needed to grow their families and create believers.

The Bible has many stories of women trying to have babies to no avail and describes their desires and suffering because they are unable to get pregnant. We see it with Sarah and Abraham in Genesis. Sarah gave her slave to Abraham so he could get her pregnant, but then Sarah gets jealous and feels great suffering after her slave gets pregnant.

In the story of Jacob and Rachel in Genesis, Rachel was unable to have children while her sister, Leah, was having babies with Jacob left and right. (Yes, Rachel and Leah were sisters married to the same man—oh, and Jacob was their cousin. I will talk more about the juicy details of this story in a later chapter.) This led to feelings of animosity and Rachel was really upset she wasn't able to give Jacob a son, so she gave her slave to him to bear children.

We also see in Hannah's story in 1 Samuel that she was unable to conceive. Her husband's other wife, Peninnah, made her feel less by saying God doesn't love Hannah or He would let her have a baby. Hannah prayed and prayed for God to allow her to conceive.

In all three of these stories, Sarah, Rachel, and Hannah eventually did get pregnant (with really amazing sons to boot), but we see their struggling in being unable to produce children as quickly and easily as others were able to. It makes sense that the Old Testament would speak of menstruation in a negative way since there was so much importance placed on having children and growing the faith which is exemplified in these stories.

This theme of perceived negativity in the Bible towards menstruation continues in the story of Adam and Eve, where we see the first struggle with shame and separation from God. Right off the bat when you read the first chapter of the Bible, Genesis, you read the story about Adam and Eve. They were the first man and woman who God created and they lived in the Garden of Eden. It's depicted as a paradise complete with everything they could ever need to live a miraculous life. Everything was fair play for them except one tree. They were warned not to eat the fruit from that one tree. Adam and Eve understood this restriction until Eve met a snake in the garden. The snake started asking questions and planting seeds of doubt in her mind. Finally, Eve succumbed to the doubt and not only ate the fruit herself, but convinced Adam to as well. After this, God banished Adam and Eve from the Garden of Eden and told them they would have to work hard for their food and Eve would suffer severe pains in childbirth. This is so kindly referred to as "the curse of Eve." Even though not all who believe in Jesus interpret Genesis this way, it is often referenced as the reason women experience pain not only in childbirth but in menstruation as well.

There is a lot of foreshadowing in the Old Testament of the coming of our saviour Jesus Christ. In Genesis, as God is reprimanding Adam and Eve, he also lays into the snake and says that he will be crushed and killed: Genesis 3:15 (NIV) "And I will put enmity between you and the woman, and between your offspring and hers; he will crush your head, and you will strike his heel." The snake represents Satan's evil and this verse proclaims that the snake (Satan) will be defeated. The Catholic church shows many depictions of Jesus' mother, Mary, stepping on the head of a snake because they believe it was Mary who crushed the snake's head while other denominations believe it was Jesus who crushed the powers of Hell. Whoever it is you believe 'crushed the snake's head' (Mary or Jesus) it's hard to argue against the truth that Jesus came and changed everything.

Jesus proclaimed the Great Commission in Matthew 28:19 (NIV) in saying, "Therefore go and make disciples of all nations, baptizing them in the name of the Father and of the Son and of the Holy Spirit." There was a shift from emphasizing creating believers solely through procreation to spreading the Word of the Lord to all nations and creating disciples from non-believers, not just having children. This was a fundamental alteration to the way in which believers created discipleship. It shifted the focus from having children and keeping the bloodline of Israel to spreading the Word and exemplifying the faith to attract followers. Therefore, the emphasis on growing families in order to spread the faith lessened along with the negative stigma of not conceiving.

With this shift, it brings me comfort knowing that menstruation, therefore, is also freed from the pressure and such a negative stigma. I'm not saying you shouldn't have as many babies as you want and create disciples through children, but it relieves that pressure—discipleship is not only on a woman's shoulders. While growing families was once the only way to grow the faith, Jesus expanded discipleship to include all nations, regardless of lineage. As a believer, you live your life and show examples of discipleship and show the non-believers what a holy woman looks like. This is enough; this is your call.

Menstruation is no longer tied to shame or impurity. Jesus came to free us from these burdens and remind us of our worth in Him. Your cycle is not a curse—it is a reflection of God's intricate design. Walk forward in confidence, knowing that your body is wonderfully made.

Dear Lord,
Help me to combat any negative feelings of shame I have toward my wonderfully created body.
Replace them with Your perfect peace that surpasses all understanding.
May Your presence bring me empowerment and confidence in my body.
Amen.

Part 2

Faith in Your Period

The Four Phases

God designed women with intention just as He created the rest of the universe. The closer you get to Him, the closer you get to optimal health. He designed your body to have a period to mark the beginning of your womanhood and to end when your body is no longer able to conceive. The menstrual cycle, like the seasons God created, has four phases. Ecclesiastes 3:1-8 (NIV) says, "There is a time for everything, and a season for every activity under the heavens: a time to be born and a time to die, a time to plant and a time to uproot, a time to kill and a time to heal, a time to tear down and a time to build, a time to weep and a time to dance, a time to scatter stones and a time to gather them, a time to embrace and a time to refrain from embracing, a time to search and a time to give up, a time to keep and a time to throw away, a time to tear and a time to mend, a time to be silent and a time to speak, a time to love and a time to hate, a time for war and a time for peace," which is such a profound way of looking at our cycles and is a great foundation for understanding how to give your body what it needs when it needs it. It's a reflection of honoring your body as you honor God and His timing.

The four phases of your menstrual cycle are: the menstrual phase, follicular phase, ovulatory phase, and luteal phase. Our menstrual cycles are cyclical like the seasons—winter, spring, summer, fall—going round and round on repeat. Just as we see in Ecclesiastes, God designed the seasons of the Earth, just as He designed the seasons of a woman's body. When we start looking at the characteristics of each of the four phases of our cycles, we see many similarities with the seasons. Winter is akin to our menstrual phase; cold, baren, low energy. Spring is aligned with the follicular phase when there is renewal and nature comes back to life as does your energy level and social life. Summer is like your ovulatory phase with super high energy, excitement, and ample social engagements. Lastly, fall mirrors your body's luteal phase when your energy starts to slow down and nature (and your body) starts to prepare for rest in another winter.

Many women see their cycles as two phases: period and no period. For most of my menstruating life, I really just thought of my cycle as having a period and not having a period. I knew my body ovulated, but never thought about that being a unique part of the cycle—it was just a piece of not having my period. It wasn't until I was in my thirties that I learned the truth: there are four distinct phases in our menstrual cycle. I had been cycling for almost twenty years before I knew this! So if you have been menstruating for a while and are just learning this now, you're in good company. I have felt so many emotions around my understanding of my body as I learn more: guilt, shame, embarrassment, confusion. But overall, I didn't know what I didn't know and now that I know—I can do better. If you are feeling any kind of way, don't beat yourself up for what you didn't know. You're doing an amazing job.

Here is a brief overview of the phases and later in the chapter we will dive deeper into how to support your body through each phase.

The easiest phase to notice is **the menstrual phase** because this is the phase when your body is bleeding. Pretty hard to miss this one! Bleeding typically lasts from days 1-7. A bleed less than four days or longer than seven days is often a sign of an imbalance, but it is not something to freak out about. Not only because stress and other factors impact your cycle, but because you are bioindividual. You are unique and your body does not have to fit in a time table. During your menstruation, your hormone levels are low and your body is going through a detoxification process.

After menstruation, you enter **the follicular phase**. This phase is typically days 8-11. Please remember that these timeframes are not exact and everyone has a different length of their phases which is why getting in tune with your body is important (more on the specifics of how to do that are in the next section on tracking your cycle). Even if in one cycle you had a follicular phase that lasted until day 11, your next cycle could vary. Take these typical day lengths with a grain of salt and do not worry if your phases are different from these timeframes. During this phase your body is releasing Follicle Stimulating Hormone to prime your egg for release and your estrogen is on the rise. When I talk about estrogen, please keep in mind that estrogen is not just one hormone, but comprises multiple estrogen hormones.

Next up is **the ovulatory phase**. Ovulation is when your egg is released, your estrogen and testosterone are dominating the hormone game, and you are your most fertile. Testosterone is usually associated as a male hormone, but women have testosterone as well; just not as high levels as males have. Ovulation typically occurs between days 12-17. Again, and I cannot stress this enough, these numbers are not exact and your body might be different than these numbers.

Lastly, right before you menstruate again, your body goes through **the luteal phase**. This is when your progesterone takes center stage and your body begins to warm. Your uterine lining is beginning to detach and the corpus luteum (a temporary endocrine organ that releases hormones) fades away. Typically, this phase is between days 18-28.

Not to sound like a total broken record or anything, but you are a bioindividual and these days are only averages. The best way to gain a better understanding of your averages is to track your period month over month for an extended period of time, like a year or more. This will help you become more familiar with your body's personal time frames with each phase. We will dive into tracking as we move on. However, pay attention to your body and watch for abnormally longer or shorter whole cycle lengths. Typically if cycles are longer than 38 days or shorter than 24, it could indicate an imbalance. I am not a doctor and I don't know your body, so always trust your gut and seek support from trusted advisors if you are concerned that something is off. Never forget that you know your body better than anyone else including any doctor. If you feel like something is amiss, don't ignore it and don't let anyone else dismiss your concern.

Tracking Your Cycles

When you are tracking your cycle, it can be easy to fall into a negative space and find everything that is wrong. While you are tracking, especially if you are doing this for the first time, I challenge you to simply be an observer. Do not impose judgment on your body. You do not have to give energy to every thought or observation you make. This process is not about changing anything or making your body feel one way or another. Just take note of how you are feeling and what is going on in your body and your life. Simply being in tune with your body is a superpower that you are capable of.

Once you feel you have an intimate relationship with your body and a better understanding of how you operate (because we ALL operate in our own ways), you can then figure out the best way you need support so that you can feel confident in your beautiful body. Here are some of my favorite ways of tracking the phases of the menstrual cycle.

Basal Body Temperature (BBT) Tracking

First, you'll need a basal body thermometer which you can pick up at a local store or online and there's a wide price range available as well. This is not something that you need to spend an arm and a leg on. These thermometers measure to the hundredth of a degree which is important because even slight changes in your temperature can indicate a new phase or shift in your hormones.

When you take your temperature, it needs to be the very first thing you do in the morning. Keep the thermometer next to your bed so you don't have to stand up or even sit up. Do not drink anything, talk, go to the bathroom. NOTHING. This has to be the very first thing you do.

17

You need to have at least three hours of consecutive sleep prior to taking your temperature as well. For instance, if at 3:00am you wake up to go to the bathroom and wake up at 5:30am to take your temperature, you have not gotten three hours of consecutive sleep. It is also best to take your temperature at the same time every morning or at least within an hour for the most accurate reading.

Why?

Anything you do that could alter your temperature needs to be avoided. These are other things that can impact your temperature:

- Time zone travel
- Daylight savings time
- Sickness
- Extreme stress
- Alcohol consumption

If you do have these things come up—and let's face it they come up—don't worry about it and just note it in your chart. If you are keeping your temperatures in an app on your phone there is usually a spot to add comments and if you use paper you can just write in the margins. As long as you are aware that a temperature change could be because of another reason than your hormones shifting, you'll have the data you need to be able to track your phases.

There are some options for recording your temperature. The first is the old school way: write it down on paper. Be sure to write down the date with the temperature and any other note you need to make (like if any of those variables listed above occurred). If you aren't into the paper option, there are many apps available where you can record your temperatures among other things such as period tracking, ovulating tracking, emotions, physical activity, etc.

*A word of caution when using apps to record your period. This technology is great and uses predictive software to estimate when you will be ovulating and get your next period. However, these are estimates, predictions, guesses. Yes, they are based on trends. Yes, some women find these to be spot on. BUT there is nothing that will replace getting in tune with your own body.

One summer, I was visiting friends and staying in their son's bedroom. Before going on the trip, I knew in my gut that I was going to get my period. My intuition was screaming at me loudly. However, I looked at my app—which I never did and knew better than to rely on—but according to my app, I had at least five days before it would come. LIES. I woke up two days later on our last morning there to a crime scene. Not only did I destroy the bottom and top sheets, but the comforter and mattress cover as well. I was beyond mortified. Not because I was embarrassed that my friends were going to find out I had my period or because I thought it was gross, but because I ruined my friend's son's bed as a guest in their home. Equal embarrassment spread throughout my body the day before when my young son snuck into the room, took my bright red lipstick out of my purse, and used it to scribble all over the same bed spread. (Kind of prophetic, don't you think?) At that point I just wanted to burn the entire bed set and buy them a new one.

My story serves as a tremendous reminder that no app or other person will ever know your body better than you. Technology is great as a tool when used properly, but your intuition—your knowledge of your own body—will always be best. Always listen to your body; even if an app tells you something different. Your body knows.

On a side note here: I learned a great trick from my midwives for washing blood! I gave birth with midwives at home and was astounded that there wasn't a trace of blood anywhere. They told me to use hydrogen peroxide on the blood, and it works like a charm. All you have to do is put it on the blood directly, it bubbles a bit, and then you wash it. I use this all the time, including when I was contemplating arson on my friend's bed set. I'm fully relieved to say that my friend reported the stains came out.

Once you have your temperatures recorded wherever you choose to record them, you'll need to know how to read them. What does it all mean?

To repeat myself for the millionth time here, your body is *your* body. I could tell you exact temperatures of what "should" be or are the average temperatures, but overall it's a bioindividual reading. Your body might naturally have a warmer base temperature than the average, so don't take these numbers to heart.

Whatever your temperatures are, they will be lower before ovulation. After ovulation, your temperature will increase. To know for sure that ovulation has occurred, your temperature should be raised for a consecutive three days by at least 2/10 of a degree. Remember, your temperature could rise due to the other factors listed above, so it's important to wait for the three days of consecutively higher temperatures to make sure you have ovulated and it wasn't just an outlier reading.

Basal Body Temperature readings are a very accurate way of knowing when you ovulate, although it is not a 100% guaranteed way of knowing. Remember that this is a fantastic way for you to know how to best support your body through each phase of your cycle.

It's important to note that the information presented here is not Natural Family Planning. These are pieces that are needed when learning about NFP, but this book is not a resource for how to conceive (or not conceive).

Cervical Fluid Tracking

Does anyone else get a little uncomfortable reading that subtitle? The best way to describe the feeling of thinking about "cervical fluid" would be with an emoji—the one with the squiggly mouth, red cheeks, one eye wide open the other closed, with one raised eyebrow. This is not a topic that comes with ease to many women, but it is a VERY accurate way of knowing which phase of your cycle you are in.

How do you track your fluid? Well, you can just look in your underwear, look at the toilet paper every time you go to the bathroom, or use your fingers. Each option works based on your own comfort. However, if you don't see any in your underwear or on your toilet paper, it's a good idea to use your fingers to get a clear picture of what your cervical fluid looks like.

Here's what your cervical fluid is telling you:
- Menstrual Phase
    - This is when you are bleeding, so this is the most obvious of the fluids.

- Follicular Phase
  - ° Your cervical fluid will start out a bit dry following your period, but then it will take on a creamy consistency. The fluid will be creamy, milky, lotiony, and white in color. It will look and feel wet.
- Ovulatory Phase
  - ° This is when your cervical fluid will almost resemble raw egg whites—it will be clear and stretch between your fingers ½ - 1 inch. When ovulating, many women experience gushes of watery sensations. The last day you experience this wet sensation before switching to dry is your day of ovulation. The shift to dry is typically abrupt and immediate after you ovulate.
- Luteal Phase
  - ° This is when your cervical fluid is sticky, tacky, pasty, and thicker. It remains thicker until your period.

When your body temperature rises is also the time when your cervical fluid gets thicker. Here's how I think of it: you know how when you heat foods up they get thicker? It is like your body heats up and "cooks" your fluids making them thicker and stickier. This is just how I think of it.

If this is your first time tracking your periods, pick one method and stick with it for a handful of cycles/months. Don't try to do everything all at once because it can overwhelm you and it's harder to get in a habit if you are doing too many new things at once. Pick one, try it out, observe your body. After some time, try out another method and decide which method you like best.

Birth Control

I do not speak highly of birth control—especially hormonal birth control—and I don't want to dwell on this topic, but it is something that needs to be addressed. This information is not meant to shame, guilt, or cause fear if you currently are on or ever have been on birth control. And if you are on birth control and decide to stop, please make sure that it is your choice. This book is not intended to be medical advice. When I write about birth control, I am not writing about condoms or other similar products. What I am referring to are the pills, injections, rings, patches, IUDs, or any artificial hormone therapy.

Not all religions or churches under the Christian umbrella agree on their stances on birth control. Some churches see every form of blocking conception as bad while others are more okay with it. Many churches see it as a way for couples to plan their family so they can have children when they are ready. Other churches see birth control as synonymous with abortion whether the conception would have occurred or not without the contraception. I am not going to dive into these views of which church preaches what because they are so contrary and politically charged. Not to mention this is not the focus of the book and that topic alone could be its own book.

Whatever your stance, I hope that you will keep an open mind as I examine how detrimental artificial hormones are to your health. Here's how I've wrestled with this as a Christian woman and coach—this isn't a judgment, but a nudge to ask questions.

The reason why I, as a Christ-following, integrative nutrition health coach specialized in hormone health, am not in support of birth control is because it absolutely wreaks havoc on our bodies.

Story time! I missed a lot of school in middle and high school because I had cramps so bad I could hardly get out of bed. If I made it to school, I would end up leaving early because I was in so much pain. On the upside, this came in handy when I wanted to get out of gym class. Don't judge me, I know I'm not the only one who has ever used my period as an excuse to get out of something. Genesis 31:34-35 shows me I'm not the only one who has used my period as an excuse. Remember back to the sisters, Leah and Rachel, who married the same man who was also their cousin? This story always makes me chuckle as I can relate to Rachel using her period to her advantage. If you're unfamiliar, the full story goes like this:

Jacob needed a wife and when he met Rachel, he knew she was the one. When he went to Rachel's father, Laban, he was told to work for seven years and then he could marry Rachel. Jacob did his time and married…LEAH! Oops. Laban played a big trick on Jacob and had his other daughter Leah marry Jacob. Jacob was not happy as you could imagine. He loved Rachel. So Laban said he could work for another seven years and marry Rachel. Done deal. Both sisters married Jacob. Now, when they were leaving Laban's house to go back to Jacob's hometown, Rachel stole Laban's precious household idols. You know what they say about a woman scorned! When Laban was trying to find his idols, Rachel played her own trick and sat on them on her horse while Laban frantically accused Jacob of taking them and searched their convoy. When she was questioned, Rachel said she had her period and couldn't stand up for her father to search. Her father, understanding what having her period meant, didn't press her to get up for him to search. She got away with theft all thanks to her period.

I am not condoning theft, lying, or trickery. Jacob eventually finds out and isn't thrilled. But even the Bible shows that sometimes your period comes in handy!

Back to my period. My PMS was out of control for years, so of course when we talked with my doctor, the first solution posed was to go on birth control. Because why not put a young woman on hormone altering drugs instead of questioning her health habits and lifestyle, right?

This was not a good choice. Did it make my monthly bleed come like clockwork? Yes. Did it make my pains subside? Yes. BUT did it give me migraines? Yes. Did it give me insanely heavy bleeds? Yes. Did it screw up my gut? Yes. Did it deplete vital nutrients from my body? Yes. Did it do more harm than good? A resounding YES.

One common misconception about your bleed while on birth control is that it is your period. It is not a period. It's referred to as a withdrawal bleed because of the crash or "withdrawal" of hormones. Why is this less than ideal for your health? Because this bleed is not due to the shedding of the lining of your uterus. Our menstrual phase is a built-in purification system, allowing the body to renew itself monthly. Just as Leviticus speaks about cleansing rituals, our bodies follow similar patterns, shedding the old to make way for the new. When your body is distracted by artificial hormones that confuse the body and block a true cleansing period, your body is not detoxing in the way God created it to.

Your body is not following natural hormone ebbs and flows with hormonal birth control. These fake hormones trick your body into thinking ovulation has already occurred, so your pituitary gland doesn't send signals to create other hormones. Which is also disturbing. Artificial hormones are not the same as naturally occurring hormones. All of your hormones are connected, so if your reproductive hormones are imbalanced, this can affect other hormones such as thyroid, insulin, serotonin, etc. Remember, every part of your body is connected.

When you begin tracking your natural cycle without artificial interventions, you will start to be able to predict when your bleed will begin. You will start to be able to read the signs in your own body and read into those signs to tell you if something could be off with your body. Our cycles are sacred and should be treated as such.

Supporting Your Body Through Phases

As I discussed earlier, your hormones fluctuate throughout the twenty-eight or so days of the menstrual cycle, so when we are supporting our bodies through each phase, that support is going to vary depending on the phase in which your body is. This is where tracking your cycle and really getting in tune with your body comes into play.

1 Corinthians 10:31 (NIV) says, "So whether you eat or drink or whatever you do, do it all for the glory of God." Taking care of your body and giving it the support it requires is more than just being some kind of health nut. Do it for the glory of God. He created your body and made no mistakes. The mistakes come from man-made problems and unnecessary interventions. Let's

take a look at what you can eat and how you can optimize your body's energy to best support your hormones during each phase of your cycle.

Menstrual Phase
You know how God created the world? He created the sun and the moon, He created land and sea, He created plants and animals, He created man and woman. After all of this work He rested. HE RESTED. And through all of His teachings, He never tells us that we must work ourselves to the brink of death in order to *earn* rest. He just tells us to rest. REST my friend! There is a time for action and there is a time for rest—just like throughout our menstrual cycles.

The seventh day in our creation story is the day for rest. The end of the week, right? When I give my workshops around cycle syncing and optimally supporting your body through the cycle, I use the bleeding phase as the first phase. Most books and courses on menstruation do the same. Apps count day 1 of your cycle on the first day of your bleed. Now, in a circle, there's really no start and end, however, I've been thinking more and more about this idea of resting on the final day and how our bodies are connected to the Bible and the amazing nature that God created. It makes more sense that our menstruation is actually the end of the cycle because it is the shedding needed to renew.

God speaks about rest all over the Bible. Besides the fact that God created the world in seven days and on the last day rested; His message to rest is littered throughout the Bible. Hebrews 4:9-10 (NIV) calls us to rest in saying, "There remains, then, a Sabbath-rest for the people of God; for anyone who enters

27

God's rest also rests from their works, just as God did from his." God is calling us to rest as a way to show we trust and obey Him. It's not out of laziness; it's out of trust and faith in the Lord.

The number seven is used throughout the Bible as a representation of rest. There are eight prayer watches that, while not directly mentioned in the Bible, stem from the concept of watchmen on walls serving an essential purpose in ancient and Biblical cities throughout the Bible such as in Isaiah 62:6 (NIV) which says, "I have posted watchmen on your walls, Jerusalem; they will never be silent day or night." The seventh watch occurs between 12:00 PM and 3:00 PM and is known as a time of rest, prayer, and seeking God's guidance. During this timeframe, Jesus was hanging on the cross bleeding for us. The seventh watch epitomizes the menstrual phase of your cycle: it's a time of rest and the time in which Jesus bled just as your body is in need of rest during your bleed.

Psalm 23 is a very popular one with many Christian songwriters giving it glory. Psalm 23:1-6 (NIV) says, "The Lord is my shepherd; I lack nothing. He makes me lie down in green pastures, he leads me beside quiet waters, he refreshes my soul. He guides me along the right paths for his name's sake. Even though I walk through the darkest valley, I will fear no evil, for you are with me; your rod and your staff, they comfort me. You prepare a table before me in the presence of my enemies. You anoint my head with oil; my cup overflows. Surely goodness and love will follow me all the days of my life, and I will dwell in the house of the Lord forever." There are so many juicy pieces to Psalm 23 in regards to placing your trust in God, but it also gives us the calm to rest. He makes you lie down in green pastures and leads you by still waters. Find the calm in Him and obey Him by resting.

Every book or website I read growing up and even while learning more during my hormone intensive course, says the first day of your cycle is marked as your first day of your bleed. This seems counterintuitive since the final day is rest, all of the hormonal shifts and ovulation need to happen prior to bleeding, and there's really this sense of finality when you get your period; not of new beginning. The only reason I can think of for using the first day of the bleed as day 1 of a cycle is that it is the easiest to detect. So in a world dictated by "science" and numbers, this comes to be day 1. However, in the world of spirituality and God's creation of nature, this is counterintuitive.

As you move through your cycle, take the number of days a certain phase should be happening with a grain of salt. Most books and websites give a range in which most women fall for the number of days phases last. What I urge all women to do is get so in tune with your body that you know what's "normal" for your body that when something is off, you know based on your own body—not some number decided by a bunch of people who don't know you.

During your cycle, as you know and saw in previous chapters, your hormones fluctuate. Unlike men who have a 24 HOUR hormonal cycle, we ladies have a 28 DAY cycle. We are not the same person at the end of our cycle as we were at the beginning. And we were not designed to be! This is not a bad thing. Just as the energy we feel from the moon is not the same during each of its phases or the energy in nature during all four seasons. We are nature and the closer we get to living in alignment with the natural energies of life, the more optimal our health outcomes are. Remember, God doesn't make mistakes. We were created to ebb and flow in our energy.

Much of the emphasis of this section on the menstrual phase is on rest because modern day women are really good at high energy. When I talk about rest, I don't mean laziness. What I mean is having increased grace with your body, light movement, saying, "no," to activities that don't support your energy, and accepting that your body relies on phases of less intensity. Our world is intense. Many wear burning the candle from both ends and doing it all as a badge of honor. Let's wear feeling fully rested as a badge of honor. My body was feeling tired, so I did some light stretching, went for a walk, read my Bible, ate some home-made deliciousness, and that was my day. It's also so important to switch the mindset that a day when that's "all you did" was a productive day and not a lazy wasted day.

Historically, during the time when the Bible was written, ancient cultures had practices where women lived together in a dwelling separate from the rest of society for the duration of their periods. These dwellings have become widely known as "red tents." While some cultures practiced this, the Bible does not mandate or even mention menstrual seclusion or the "red tents," it's only found in historical documents from the time.

You have probably heard the stories of women going to the "red tent" during their periods, if not, now you have! Many in the secular world who view the Bible as oppressive to women see this practice as unjust, sexist, and demeaning. But what if this practice wasn't founded in patriarchy and instead was based on what is best for a woman's cycle even if it isn't a Biblical practice? Instead of viewing menstruation as something to be hidden away, the Bible—especially the New Testament with Jesus' teaching—shows that a woman's body is part of God's intentional design, to be honored and embraced. So perhaps the idea of the red tent in regards to fulfilling rest is a practice that honors women, not a practice to hide women from society.

During your period your body is not best equipped for work and socialization. Energy levels are low thanks to the giant drop in estrogen.

We need to be more focused on resting our bodies during our periods and less focused on being able to conquer the world. It's very advanced that we ladies can wear a cup, disc, or a tampon and go master a triathlon, but you are defying your body's natural energy flow and aren't supporting it when you partake in these events during your period. Of course I understand that large events like this cannot simply be rescheduled to fit your menstrual cycle and those who are dedicated to these events don't have much of a choice sometimes, but if you do have a choice, it is always best to do what supports your body.

Again, when I talk about resting your body, I'm not suggesting you live a sedentary existence for a week. No, no, no. There are many forms of light movement you can do to keep active, but still allow rest. If you are taking work-out classes opt for the easier modifications, go on walks, or just simply stretch. These lighter movements allow your body to focus on its detoxing and healing work it's doing during your period.

During this phase, your body is undergoing a lot of change and doing a lot of work. You might be feeling high energy based on various factors, but keep in mind that your body is at work. This is a great time to move with ease and take more breaks. Give yourself ample grace during your menstrual phase.

Period Hygiene

When you get your period, consider letting your body free bleed as much as possible. You can use a cotton disposable or reusable pad if you can do a free bleed. Why does this matter? There are fewer issues that can arise and it's more natural for your body. You've probably learned that when you use a tampon, you need to be careful not to leave it in too long because you can end up with TSS (toxic shock syndrome). Tampons are more often than not bleached to make the cotton white and therefore expose a very sensitive and absorbent part of the body to bleach along with a whole slew of other chemicals used to make tampons.

When you are inserting really anything into your vagina, it's important hygiene to wash your hands before and after doing so. Why? Your vagina is a very absorbent sponge so whatever is on your hands is quickly and easily absorbed. If you just eliminated your bowels, think of what you just touched and are now contaminating your sensitive, absorbent vagina with. It's very good practice to wash your hands with a toxin-free soap before and after.

In the following table are some pros and cons regarding feminine care products. These are general pros and cons to support your thinking process if you are considering changing up your hygiene routine. For most of my womanhood, I received negative messages from other women about free bleeding and using pads. My own journey took me from using tampons and disposable pads to using a disc and reusable pads for a number of various reasons from what my body was being exposed to, comfort, and expense. Take the information, let it marinate a bit, and make your own choice. What is important to one woman is not important to another.

Pros and Cons of Feminine Hygiene Products

Product	Pros	Cons
Reusable Pads (Organic cotton and unbleached)	• Less garbage in the landfill • Exposed to fewer chemicals • Free bleed • Many women experience fewer and less intense cramping • Long-term cost	• Cleaning • Availability if you weren't prepared and not home • Don't prevent odors • Upfront cost
Disposable Pads (Organic and non-organic)	• Available in a pinch • Don't have to wash • Many women experience fewer and less intense cramping • Upfront cost	• Chemical exposure • Don't prevent odors • End up in landfills • Long-term cost
Tampons (Organic and non-organic)	• Available in a pinch • Disposable • Upfront cost • Prevent odors	• Chemical exposure • Risk of TSS (Toxic Shock Syndrome) • End up in landfills or water facilities • Dry out vagina • Long-term costs
Menstrual Cups (Medical Grade Silicone)	• Less garbage in landfill • Exposed to fewer chemicals • Many women experience fewer and less intense cramping • Long-term cost	• Sizing • Take out to empty • Cleaning • Availability—needs to be boiled before first use • Upfront cost
Discs (Medical Grade Silicone)	• Less garbage in landfill • Exposed to fewer chemicals • Many women experience fewer and less intense cramping • Empties when urinating or eliminating bowels • Disposable options available • Long-term cost	• Cleaning • Availability—needs to be boiled before first use (reusable only) • Upfront cost
Absorbent Underwear	• Less garbage in landfill • Comfort • Many women experience fewer and less intense cramping • Long-term cost	• Chemical exposure in various brands • Cleaning • Availability in a pinch • Upfront cost

Supportive Foods

When you're putting together your meal plan, it's extra important to think about blood sugar balancing foods. Even though
it's important to be aware of balancing blood sugar throughout
your entire cycle, it's worth a little extra focus during your bleed.
Protein is essential. It's important to always be aware of your
protein. Protein can come in a vegetarian/vegan diet, however,
if you're not consuming meat or animal products, it is essential to supplement with B12 and if you're eating vegan, supple-
menting not only with B12, but also vitamin D, and calcium.
I'm not trying to convince anyone to not be vegetarian or vegan,
however, many pill form supplements are not as bioavailable as
eating a real source (like a steak). Just keep this in mind when you
are looking at how you eat.

Iron-rich foods are key during your menstrual phase. Think
about it: you're bleeding and iron is a key nutrient in blood. So
replenishing your iron stores using real foods is a pretty good
idea. I would be very careful with iron supplements, though.
Real food is the best source of nutrients. Foods that are iron rich
include grass-fed beef, eggs, and spinach. Nutrient density can
be determined by the quality of the food, so look for organic,
grass-fed and regeneratively farmed (beef), or pasture-raised
(chicken/eggs).

Bone broth is gold. I can't sing its praises enough. Whenever I
think of a healing meal, I think of chicken and veggie soup with
bone broth. We see it in movies, read about it in books, and experience it firsthand—when people get sick, they eat soup. You are
not sick when you have your period, but when you're feeling low
energy, maybe a bit crampy or bloated, feeling a bit of an ick—a

nice bone broth soup is clutch. I will warm up a cup or two on my stove and drink beef bone broth straight.

Why is bone broth so healing? Well, real bone broth is full of vitamins and nutrients from the bones as well as gelatin. Gelatin does wonders in healing the gut and supporting proper functions. If you're buying a bone broth from the store, be sure to look for organic, grass-fed, pasture-raised/regeneratively farmed beef. Some may have added gelatin, and when you cool it, you should be able to see the thick gelatin. I will purposely not suggest a specific brand because brands, unfortunately, can change their recipes—especially if they're bought out—and some simply go out of business. If you want to make some on your own, there are a million recipes online.

Here's one recipe you can use to make your own beef bone broth:
Ingredients:
-3 to 4 pounds of mixed beef bones, short ribs, oxtails, knuckles, and neck bones (check out local butchers who offer grass-fed, organic, regenerative farming types of meats)
-1 tablespoon olive or avocado oil (don't use seed oils such as canola, corn, sunflower, safflower, soy, etc. These are xeno-estrogens and are considered endocrine disruptors.)
-2 medium carrots
-3 celery stalks
-2 medium yellow onions
-2 tablespoons cider vinegar
-1 bay leaf
- water
* I also suggest eating as organic as you possibly can. When your body isn't inundated by detoxing, it can have the energy to use for supporting hormones and other vital functions.

Instructions:

1. Preheat your oven to 400F. While the oven is warming up, place your beef bones in a single layer on a baking tray and drizzle with oil.

2. Roast the beef bones for 30 minutes on each side. While the bones are roasting, prepare your vegetables by cutting them up into chunks.

3. Once the bones are ready, combine all the ingredients in a slow cooker or a large stockpot. Cover with water so everything is immersed, and add 2 tablespoons of apple cider vinegar.

4. Put on the lid and turn the stockpot to high setting. Once it reaches a rapid simmer, lower the setting to low, and simmer for 12-24 hours. Check occasionally to top off with water as needed.

5. After it's done simmering, strain the vegetables and bones. Most of the nutrients will have been extracted, so you can discard or compost the ingredients. Pour the broth into mason jars and store in the fridge.

When you're ready to consume, you can reheat it and drink it straight or add it to a soup, rice, noodles, almost anything you might cook in water you can cook in bone broth. Don't worry about the fat that will harden on the top. That is gold! Just warm it up, stir it in, and enjoy!

Remember, your menstrual phase is like your internal winter. Low energy and cold. These warming foods can be healing not only for your body, but for your soul as well.

Prayer for your menstrual cycle:

Jesus,
This is my time to slow down. My body is tired and I feel it deep in my bones. Thank you for designing me with cycles of renewal, not constant striving.
Help me to let go of the guilt I feel when I need rest.
I don't want to push through or pretend like I'm fine when I'm not. I want to honor the way You made me.
This blood I shed each month used to make me feel gross or broken. But now I see it's part of Your rhythm. It's a holy reset.
Be near to me in this quiet space. Help me hear You in the stillness. Thank You for calling me to rest, not because I've earned it—but because You love me.
Amen.

Follicular Phase

As this is the phase that resembles spring, it is a reawakening of the body and energy. This is the phase to increase your intensity in your workouts. As your estrogen begins to rise again, your body is getting primed for higher energy activities. During your follicular phase, you'll be ready for the high intensity work-outs. This is the time for triathlon training! It's a great time to say, "Yes!" to all of the social events.

Remember how in the beginning of time there was only Adam and Eve? And they were responsible for creating an entire population? Well, God had a plan for this. He designed our female bodies to be exciting, energetic, and social during the time we are primed for procreation and grumpy and irritable during the time we are not because who would want to create more humans with someone who is moody and irritable? God is one brilliant creator!

Again, the follicular phase presents an increase in energy resulting in it being a great time to get your creative juices flowing, brainstorm, make plans, go hiking, work up a sweat, and strength train.

Making plans always makes me chuckle a bit and think of the old adage that if you want to hear God laugh, tell Him your plans. It's not to suggest you move through life without direction, but more so to trust that God has great plans for you and if the plan you're creating isn't the one He has for you, do not fear. Trust it will be okay.

Psalm 20:4 (NIV) says "May he give you the desire of your heart and make all your plans succeed." This verse is not suggesting that your plans succeed no matter what the plan is. What this is really talking about is in the first part about the desire of your heart—the desire of loving God, doing His work, following the example of Jesus. These aren't just desires of man, these are desires of heart—love—God.

Supportive Foods
During your follicular phase your estrogen is rising, so the focus here is on foods that support estrogen. It's a great time to focus on your high quality fats such as grass-fed organic butter or avocado oil. Fat has gotten a really bad reputation, but the high quality fats are insanely essential in your diet. Keep in mind that seed oils such as canola, corn, sunflower, safflower, soy, etc. are xeno-estrogens and are considered endocrine disruptors. In other words, they mimic estrogen and therefore confuse your body.

Other yummy foods to consider during this phase are pomegranates, pumpkin seeds, flax seeds, or sprouted beans. Sprouted beans and grains are generally easier on your digestive system and therefore more ideal.

Here's the recipe for a lovely pear, pomegranate, and pumpkin seed salad with poppyseed dressing:

Ingredients:

Salad:
-8oz spinach or other favorite greens
-2 bartlett pears
-⅔ cup pomegranate seeds
-⅓ cup pumpkin seeds
-3 chopped dates
-⅓ cup slivered almonds
-3oz feta or goat cheese crumble

Dressing:
-½ cup greek yogurt, plain, whole
-⅓ cup apple cider vinegar
-2 Tbsp honey - more to taste
-1 Tbsp poppy seeds
-1 tsp garlic powder
-2 tsp onion powder
-½ tsp Celtic sea salt
-¼ tsp black pepper

Instructions:
1. Chop up all salad ingredients and combine gently in a bowl.
2. Whisk together all dressing ingredients in a separate bowl.
3. Drizzle desired amount of dressing over salad.

You could add a protein like some grilled chicken on top of the salad or it could be the side to any main course. Enjoy!

Prayer for Follicular Phase:

> *Hey God,*
> *I feel a shift today—lighter, brighter, more alive. There's energy stir-*
> *ring in me again. I can feel the possibilities.*
> *Thank You for this new beginning. For hormones that rise, for thoughts*
> *that spark, for hope that returns after the slump.*
> *In this phase when I want to say yes to everything, remind me that my*
> *plans are safe in Your hands.*
> *Let my creativity be rooted in You.*
> *Let my confidence reflect You—not just what my body can do, but who*
> *You say I am.*
> *And when I forget, when I overdo it or lose direction, gently bring me*
> *back to Your purpose.*
> *Amen.*

Ovulatory Phase

Hello gorgeous! This is the phase that resembles summer and is your highest energy phase. Whenever I visualize the energy of the ovulatory phase, I imagine it like in 2 Samuel 6:14-22 when King David was dancing through the streets for the Lord as the house of Israel brought up the ark and trumpets played. This is a time of celebration in your body! You're at your peak level of estrogen and primed for your highest energy activities. It's your time to maximize your own potential—and dance through the streets!

Your estrogen is at its peak during ovulation, but you are about to have a major crash as your progesterone takes over after ovulation. In order to prepare yourself for this sharp decline in estrogen, it's important to support your body in detoxification so your body can detox the excess estrogen.

It's very common for women in our modern society to have high estrogen, otherwise called estrogen dominance. It's estimated that roughly 72% of women experience estrogen dominance, so this detox is crucial. Does this percentage shock you? It doesn't shock me. Let's think about the liver. It is a major detox organ that gets overburdened by a lot of toxins in our body. If you're using personal care products full of toxins, eating foods that are processed and grown with toxins, drinking alcohol, cleaning your house with chlorine/bleach-based products, or any other toxins in our environment, your liver is prioritizing those toxins that are most poisonous and the other toxins (or in this case hormones) are being put to the back burner. So if your body is going to choose between detoxing that glass of wine you had at dinner or your excess estrogen, it's going to detox the alcohol first.

This is why toxic load matters.

Besides lowering your toxic load and making swaps in your products for low-tox or toxin-free products, there are some foods that you can incorporate into your meal planning to support your liver in detoxification.

Cruciferous veggies such as brussels sprouts, kale, cabbage, turnips, or broccoli are very supportive in detoxification. I love beets, too. It's a root vegetable and some ways of preparing them are better than others. Pickled beets have grown on me, but my favorite way to prepare beets is to roast them. I slice them up, lay them in a single layer on a baking sheet, spray them heavily with avocado oil or put a dollop of grass-fed ghee (a clarified butter) on each piece, and sprinkle them with Celtic sea salt and onion powder. I bake at 425 F for about 20 minutes. Chef's kiss. I like to do broccoli this way sometimes on the same baking sheet as beets. So good.

Another delicious dish that supports liver detox is raw carrot salad. Many health coaches even suggest women eat raw carrot salad daily considering the high percentage of women who have estrogen dominance.

Here's how I make mine:
-1-2 carrots shredded
-1 tsp avocado oil
-1tsp apple cider vinegar
-1 tsp honey or to taste
-a pinch of Celtic sea salt

I often shred up a bunch of carrots and then take my daily serving out to mix with the dressing.

Prayer for your Ovulatory Phase:

Dear Lord,
I feel radiant right now. Thank You for this high-energy, high-capacity season in my cycle.
I feel magnetic—like I want to love hard, laugh loud, connect deeply. It's wild how You built all of this into me - how my body reflects the same joy I imagine You had when You created the world.
Help me use this energy well. Let it not just be for performance or perfection but for celebration, generosity, and love.
Keep me grounded in You, even when I'm soaring.
Thank You for the beauty of this phase. Let me walk through it fully alive and anchored in You.
Amen.

Luteal Phase

Lastly, before you begin menstruating again, you have your luteal phase. This phase gets the worst reputation of all the phases because of those dreaded three letters: PMS. Many women experience premenstrual syndrome (PMS) during this time to varying degrees. This can include symptoms such as mood swings, irritability, depressed feelings, anxiety, heightened emotions, fatigue, trouble sleeping, bloating, cramping, breast tenderness, headaches, spotty skin, greasy hair, or changes in appetite and food cravings. Some women experience these symptoms severely, causing them to miss out on activities, and others don't experience these symptoms at all.

If you are experiencing intense PMS symptoms, you might view this phase with dread. You might even liken it to how Jesus was beaten and tortured before He bled on the cross and you might start to just accept it as something that you must suffer through as a part of being a woman. In contrast if you do not experience these symptoms or experience a very mild version of PMS, you probably think nothing of this phase.

PMS is often blamed on hormones. Estrogen plummets and progesterone takes center stage as the lead hormone. Your body's energy during this phase is a slow taper as your progesterone rises. This phase, energy-wise, can really be split into halves. The first half is still riding high from ovulation, but it's a really good time to get odds and ends wrapped up. It's somewhat of a nesting period to finish up the to-do list so you can focus on resting during your period. You will still have the energy to do the more intense versions of movement, however, now is not the time to push yourself to beat your PRs.

I like to think of the second half as my bedtime routine phase. That time to pick up the last remaining dishes from the day, wash my face, brush my teeth, take out my contacts, put on pajamas. This is the wind down time. You can start going to bed at an earlier time to get on top of that extra sleepiness your body could experience during your period as this second half is often when women start to show signs of PMS.

This can be hard for some to accept, but PMS is not normal. It is common. Being common does not mean it is something that "should" be happening. When you were a young lady learning about the changes your body was about to go through, do you remember learning that PMS was due to a lifestyle that was not suited for your body? Did you learn all the natural ways you could prevent PMS and not just how to tame the symptoms once they arose? Did you learn that PMS is a sign that your body needs nourishment?

I certainly did not.

The lesson I received on PMS can be summed up as: take pills and put heat on your stomach.

I taught fourth grade for part of my public school teaching career which was the year of "the talk." All of the girls and female teachers gathered in one classroom while the boys did the same in another. Each room received a lesson about what to expect as their bodies were changing. I can attest from personal experience that this lesson hasn't changed.

What's worse is that the birth control pill is marketed as a way to prevent PMS symptoms. As discussed earlier, birth control does far more harm than good, especially when there are a multitude of natural options that will not impede your health.

The Book of Job in the Bible inculcates lessons about pain, suffering, praise to God, supporting friends, and understanding blame, among many others. Job was a man who had it all: a loving wife, children he doted over, wealth, and abundance. He was respected in his village and did what was right in the eyes of God. In Job, Satan talks with God and it is decided that Satan has God's permission to test Job's loyalty and faith in God. Throughout the first couple chapters, Job loses everything. His wealth and abundance are taken. His children perish. His health deteriorates as boils consume every inch of his skin. He is in a living nightmare—yet praises God anyway.

In his time of need, three of his friends come over to comfort him. Throughout most of the rest of The Book of Job is a conversation between Job and his friends. In the beginning of their visit, it seems they are loving friends, crying with Job and sitting in silence, but then they start talking and adding insult to injury. The friends start blaming Job for his misfortunes saying he must have done something to anger God.

Job 33:19-26 (NIV) shows a piece of what was discussed when Elihu, a younger man listening to Job and his friends, says, "Or someone may be chastened on a bed of pain with constant distress in their bones, so that their body finds food repulsive and their soul loathes the choicest meal. Their flesh wastes away to nothing, and their bones, once hidden, now stick out. They draw near to the pit, and their life to the messengers of death. Yet if there is an angel at their side, a messenger, one out of a thousand, sent to tell them how to be upright, and he is gracious to that person and says to God, 'Spare them from going down to the pit; I have found a ransom for them—let their flesh be renewed like a child's; let them be restored as in the days of their youth'—then that person can pray to God and find favor with him, they will see God's face and shout for joy; he will restore them to full well-being." Elihu is warning him to find favor with God, that surely he did something to make God mad and afflict him with such agony."

God was not punishing Job. He always loved Job and was with him through all of it. When your body is expressing symptoms (PMS or otherwise) you are not being punished just as Job was not being punished. It is not a time to curse the Lord and lament why he did this to you. These symptoms are your body's safe-guards to help you get closer to God! They're to support the lifestyle that honors God; not to punish you. Take a deep breath and remember your gracious and loving God is always in control. Suffering is not the punishment, it serves as a reminder of the purposes of the gospel in your life.

God doesn't call us to make life easy. He calls us to do the hard things. To go through the fire and be refined by God. Let your monthly pains be a guide to Him and to living by His ways.

God is not communicating using PMS to punish you or because He doesn't love you. He is telling you that something in the way you live is not honoring Him. PMS is saying you need to make some changes to how you are nourishing your body. This is a blessing. God made many built-in health barometers; one of which is the luteal phase. Symptoms aren't always pleasant, but they're telling you something about the bigger picture of your health. Listen to your body instead of getting frustrated with the symptoms. Take a deep breath and observe your rhythm.

When you wake up in the morning, the question to ask should not be: "What can I do today to lower the number I see on my scale?" It should not be: "What can I do for ME today?" The real question that should guide your day and reflect your health is: "What can I do to honor God?"

Is ingesting poison honoring God? Is watching the news and stressing yourself out over matters out of your control honoring God? Is giving up honoring God? Is vanity honoring God?

Preventing pain through honoring God is as simple as giving your body what it needs: prayer, rest, real food, movement, connection to others and nature, and a grateful mindset. It's moving through your day with God first and asking yourself before you make any decision: does this honor God? Would God want me to eat this or say this or do this or use this?

Supportive Foods
During this time, you'll want to focus on incorporating progesterone supporting foods into your menu. These foods are focused on vitamins and minerals. When I speak about these nutrients, I want you to focus on real, whole foods that are high in these vitamins and minerals and not run out to the store to buy some pill form supplements. I think that just like any other pharmaceutical product, our modern society is very fixated on taking a pill to fix the issue whether it's a harsh pharma product or a supplement. Real, whole foods are always going to give you a more bioavailable nutrient, meaning it is more easily absorbed into the

body for it to utilize. It doesn't pay to spend a ton of money on a nutrient that isn't being properly absorbed into your body, right?

Foods high in magnesium, to start. Honestly, the best way to get natural magnesium is Celtic sea salt. I buy the large grain and take a few grains in the morning and wash it down with a glass of water. Leafy greens are another way to incorporate more magnesium into your menu. This is not a food, but magnesium lotion or gel is another great way to absorb magnesium into your body. During the luteal phase is often when women begin to experience PMS and cramping. Magnesium aids in stabilizing your mood and is great for muscle cramping.

Vitamin B6 is emphasized during this phase, so incorporating foods such as avocado, eggs, and banana into your menu is great. One of my favorite breakfasts is a slice of sourdough with avocado and a fried egg or two on top. If I'm feeling fancy, I like to add some pickled onion or a feta or goat cheese crumble on top. I season with Celtic sea salt, onion powder, and black pepper. I'll take a banana with peanut butter on the side. Mmmm!

Vitamin C is something that a lot of people turn to supplements for. But you don't have to! Most people think of oranges when they think of vitamin C. I'll never forget my reaction when I learned that cauliflower actually has more vitamin C in it than an orange. It was a bit of awe and shock. Citrus is still a great option, but cauliflower is an option for those who aren't citrus women. Another great option is camu camu. You can get this as a powder and only a teaspoon contains 760% of your daily value of vitamin C. I take mine in a variety of ways. Sometimes I just stir it into water, I add it to a smoothie, or I make an electrolyte drink.

Here's my favorite electrolyte drink recipe:
-12 oz organic coconut water (make sure the only ingredient is coconut water)
-1 tsp camu camu powder
-¼ tsp Celtic sea salt
-1 tsp maple syrup - or to taste
-1 tbsp lemon juice

I combine the camu camu, salt, syrup, and lemon juice first with a frother. Then pour the coconut water in, stir, and enjoy!

Lastly, zinc helps support progesterone which can be consumed in many foods, some of which include red meat such as beef or lamb. Oysters are total zinc bombs and other shellfish such as crab, shrimp, and mussels are high as well, but not as high in zinc as oysters. Leviticus 11 tells us that these sea creatures are unclean and not fit to be eaten, so if this is something you consider when eating, try the other foods high in zinc. Legumes such as lentils, beans, peanuts, and chickpeas are sources of zinc. Nuts such as pine nuts, cashews, almonds, dairy, and eggs are also nice sources of zinc.

Prayer for your Luteal Phase:

God,
This phase often feels like a personal battle. I get moody. Tired. My fuse is short, and the world feels too loud.
But I don't want to fight what You created. I want to work with it.
Help me embrace this time as sacred—not shameful.
Let me prepare—not panic.
Let me reflect—not spiral.

This is the bedtime of my cycle. Help me put things in order, tie up loose ends, and rest in the knowledge that I am held—even when I feel off.

Even if I cry over something silly or want to scream over dishes in the sink, help me be kind to myself and others.

Help me to trust that You're still in this, still in me.

Thank You for Your patience, Your grace, and Your steady love.

Amen.

Part 3

Faith-Based Health

Faith-based health starts with having faith. Faith in God, faith in Jesus, faith in your body. It is focused on integrative and holistic health through getting back to nature and using what God gave us to heal and survive. It's about limiting toxin exposure, mitigating stress, and cultivating a mindset of joy and peace.

If you have the mindset that your body is broken and that you can't be healthy on your own, you are what you think. If you think you're broken; you're broken. If you think your body needs some support but it is strong, intelligent, and capable of healing on its own; it will. God designed you in His image and created you to be resilient. He did not make a mistake when He created you. Please never forget that. Your body is so immaculately intelligent. It not only goes through a menstrual cycle every month, but it heals all by itself, has the capability to grow a new human, and filters toxins. All of this is done without needing to tell your body what to do.

Before you dive into faith-based health, remember all of the information is suggestion. None of the information in this book is medical advice. I do hold credentials in integrative nutrition health coaching and am specialized in hormones, but no one knows more about your body than you. My credentials are not specific to your unique bio-individuality. They simply mean I can offer you support in finding what works for you. Even a person with a million credentials doesn't know your body better than you. If you read a suggestion and your God-given intuition is telling you not to do it—don't do it. Take back your power from any perceived authority, give it to the One true authority through prayer, and make the right choice FOR YOU.

God has the ultimate authority over you, then you, then everyone else. The lies that tell you anyone else has authority over you have become very loud and are repeated constantly making it easy to believe them. Quiet those lies with God. Take your power back with prayer.

Faith in God and Your Body
I have a sign above my bed that I read multiple times a day that is a great reminder of putting my faith where it belongs. It says, "Give it to God and go to sleep." That's what God wants us to do. It's not easy to do and it takes a lot of practice. I'm not perfect at it. There are nights when the stress is so high and even though I pray and say I'm giving it to God, it still keeps me up at night. The chapter about the menstrual phase of the cycle is very heavy on the importance of rest. Like I said before, our society is very good at rushing. Productivity is the highest standard of merit. Being busy is the standard of achievement. However, the more you slow down, the closer to God you grow, the more you will see that all of the go, go, go is only taking you away from your faith. The hustle and bustle

is just a distraction from what's really important—giving it to God and not worrying.

The Bible gives many examples of people putting all of their faith in the hands of God. In Daniel 6, Daniel, who was a respected administrator to King Darius, was set up and betrayed by fellow administrators. The other administrators were jealous of Daniel, so they set him up to be killed. They convinced the king to make a decree that for thirty days, anyone who prays to any god or human being other than Darius shall be thrown in the lions' den. They knew that Daniel was faithful to the one true God and prayed to Him. They knew when he would be praying, so they went to him during his prayer time and tattled on him to the King. Having no other option, the king threw Daniel in the lions' den as punishment for praying to God and not to him. In the lions' den, Daniel didn't take matters into his own hands. He didn't try to make a deal with King Darius to get himself out or acquiesce to the king's demands to worship him. He didn't fight the lions. He gave all of his faith to God. Here's what Daniel tells the king the next morning in Daniel 6:22-23 (NIV), "'My God sent his angel, and he shut the mouths of the lions. They have not hurt me, because I was found innocent in his sight. Nor have I ever done any wrong before you, Your Majesty.' The king was overjoyed and gave orders to lift Daniel out of the den. And when Daniel was lifted from the den no wound was found on him, because he had trusted in his God." Daniel prayed and he slept in the lions' den. It says that he was unharmed by the lions because of God's protection which is interpreted as a peaceful state such as sleep. How many "lions' dens" have you been in that you have just prayed and slept through? Wow, what a deep faith Daniel had to leave that fear to God. He literally gave it to God and went to sleep.

When Jesus was in a boat with His disciples crossing the Sea of Galilee, a raging storm came upon them. The boat was taking on water from the waves crashing over the sides and panic spread across the disciples. What did Jesus do? He didn't freak out and didn't start bailing water out of the boat. He didn't start yelling orders to the others in the boat. This is what happened according to Mark 4:37-41 (NIV), "A furious squall came up, and the waves broke over the boat, so that it was nearly swamped. Jesus was in the stern, sleeping on a cushion. The disciples woke him and said to him, 'Teacher, don't you care if we drown?' He got up, rebuked the wind and said to the waves, 'Quiet! Be still!' Then the wind died down and it was completely calm. He said to His disciples, 'Why are you so afraid? Do you still have no faith?' They were terrified and asked each other, 'Who is this? Even the wind and the waves obey him!'" In the midst of a raging sea and probably in a close to sinking boat, Jesus SLEPT! I can almost hear Jesus at the end firmly admonishing the disciples like children who just woke up their parents telling them to have faith and let Him sleep. Jesus had such a firm faith in God's plan for His life that He slept through danger when others were afraid for their lives.

Peter found himself being arrested and put in prison by King Herod. Before Peter's arrest, King Herod had put James to death for being a follower of Jesus and all the Jews were happy. They did not believe that Jesus was who he said he was, so they were delighted to learn of James' execution. Acts 12:5-7 (NIV) says, "So Peter was kept in prison, but the church was earnestly praying to God for him. The night before Herod was to bring him to trial, Peter was sleeping between two soldiers, bound with two chains, and sentries stood guard at the entrance. Suddenly, an angel of the Lord appeared and a light shone in the cell. He struck Peter on the side and woke him up. 'Quick, get up!' he said, and the chains fell off Peter's wrists." Peter's faith was so steadfast that even the night before his trial, which would undoubtedly find him guilty and not be a fair trial no matter what, he slept. He gave it to God and went to sleep.

King David is another great example of someone who put his faith in the hands of God. King David had many wives and many children. His daughter, Tamar, was raped by his son (Tamar's half-brother) Amnon. Tamar's older brother, Absalom, took her in and was outraged by their half-brother, Amnon. After some planning, Absalom murdered Amnon in revenge for his sister. Their father, King David, was furious and Absalom fled. Long story short: eventually Absalom was welcomed back to the city although King David didn't want to see him. Absalom won the hearts of the Israelites and rebelled against King David to over-throw him as king of Israel. In order to save his own life, King David packed up his household and fled. His son along with tens of thousands of his enemies were threatening his throne, life, and legacy. King David didn't spend time fretting over battle plans. He didn't take it into his own hands. King David wrote Psalm 3:5-6 (NIV) about his time fleeing from his son and said, "I lie down and sleep; I wake again, because the Lord sustains me. I will not fear though tens of thousands assail me on every side." HE SLEPT! His life was being threatened by his own flesh and blood and he handed his worry, anxiety, and fear over to God. AND HE SLEPT.

In case those examples weren't enough, Psalm 4:8 (NIV) says, "In peace I will lie down and sleep, for you alone, Lord, make me dwell in safety." Our lives are in God's hands. He's got this. He alone is your protection and savior.

God created the world and everything in it. He didn't create man and then consider what humans would need to live. He created nature and then created humans with what He already created in mind. Everything created by God is symbiotic meaning everything relies on everything else to survive. The great circle of life. The food web. Everything is connected just as all of our pieces of our body are connected. You can't intervene in one part of your body without it affecting every other part of your body. Just as you can't intervene in one part of nature without it affecting every other part of nature. Romans 1:20 (NIV) says, "For since the creation of the world God's invisible qualities— his eternal power and divine nature—have been clearly seen, being understood from what has been made, so that people are without excuse." You can see God's divine power in nature and God takes care of us. So why wouldn't nature take care of us? I'm a firm believer that health comes from being in harmony with God and nature.

Health does not have to be challenging. It does not have to be expensive. And it definitely does not come from another person.

It comes from within.

It comes from your creator; God.

It comes from the nature that God made for you.

Using Nature for Health
Grounding
When you are heading outside, consider taking your shoes off and frolic in the grass for a while. This is called grounding or earthing and is so incredibly simple. I live in the frozen tundra,

so there are some days when all the grass is covered by snow and ice or the temperatures are in the negative degrees, but you can bet I am still getting outside barefoot on days that I can see a spot of grass or the temps are in the positive integers. If you live in an area where it's either too hot or too cold for you to feel comfortable going outside barefoot, there are some other things you can do.

Sure, you could buy a grounding mat. These mats use a technology that taps into the grounding that is already in your house's electrical outlets. However, these mats are typically made out of synthetic, petroleum-based materials so is this really the greatest thing to be exposing your body to? It seems counterintuitive, but it is an option.

Or you could go outside and either stay bundled up if it's cold or keep your shoes on if it's too hot and go and touch a tree— or go wild and give it a big hug. If you're wearing mittens or gloves, it's best to take these off for you to get direct connection to the tree. Doing this, you're directly tapping into the earth because the roots of the tree are down inside the earth acting as a grounding rod.

Another option you could consider is simply taking a copper wire that is long enough to reach from outside to inside your house. Stick one end of the long copper wire into the ground outside and take the other side into the house with you. Then you hold onto the copper wire. This is another form of grounding. You don't need the latest and greatest gadget in order to do what's best for your health.

God calls us to protect and cherish the earth, he gave us dominion over the earth in Genesis, and in turn the earth provides for us! When we place our feet on the earth, we reap many benefits such as reducing inflammation, improving sleep, enhancing mood, reducing pain, lowering blood pressure, improving heart health, speeding up wound healing, enhancing immune function, improving energy levels, improving digestion, reducing anxiety, improving cognitive function, and reducing risk of certain cancers. WHOAH! What?! That list is pretty remarkable, don't you think? How does this all work? We are electrically charged beings and with that, we build up electrical charges in our bodies. When we ground or earth, we are offloading the excess electrical charges from our bodies to dissipate by absorbing the negative electrons to balance our charge. Just like how our electrical outlets in our homes need a grounding line, our bodies do, too. It's wild how something so simple (and FREE!) can have such huge impacts on your health.

Negative Ions
You have probably heard the metaphor from the Bible calling you to dance in the rain. Which is referring to seeing the joy in life even in dark times. But have you ever actually danced in the rain? Have you ever seen a perfectly beautiful rain with the sun still shining and feel drawn to it? Dancing in the rain or even just being near water: the ocean, a lake, stream, waterfall, all of these have the same effects as grounding/earthing. The falling rain, crashing waves, or cascading waters also create negative ions which boost mood, reduce stress, improve sleep, enhance energy levels, etc, etc. In the case of water, though, you can also reap these benefits by breathing in the air near the moving water. That fresh smell after a rain? Can health really be this easy? Yes. Yes it can.

Sunlight

The sun has been demonized and we have been lied to about it. Why would God have created the sun if it only killed us? Why would he have created humans if they would be killed by His earlier creation—the sun? Either way you ask the question it doesn't make sense. Sun burns are rough when you are in the sun for too long, but you know what else is detrimental to your health? Not getting adequate amounts of sun rays absorbed into your skin. Sun deprivation causes issues such as vitamin D deficiency, disrupted circadian rhythm or sleep, mood swings, weakened immune system, anxiety, depression, and many others. You might think that you are outside a lot and get lots of sun. But if you are getting sun with any sort of sunscreen, you are actually blocking beneficial rays from your skin. You can still get a tan, but you aren't reaping the benefits. Leave the sunscreen in the tube and get undisturbed sunlight on your skin. If this makes you uncomfortable or you burn easily, set some time to get undisturbed sun for an amount of time that you feel comfortable with and then put on thin layers, or seek a shady spot. While you're at it: ditch the sunglasses, too. Your eyeballs need light to be healthy, too, so try to go outside and spend some time without sunglasses. It's pretty cool that you can get health benefits FOR FREE just by going outside.

Sweat

Sweating can be gross. No one likes to raise their arms and see a sweat stain or raise their arm and have a gust of body odor fan out. Eww. BUT sweating is an essential component of your detox pathways for your body. Use a deodorant, not an antiperspirant, for odor protection while allowing your body to sweat it out. Look for deodorants with the fewest, and REAL, natural ingredients. If you are noticing strong odors from your armpits, this can be caused by your body needing to detox. A great way to support your 'pits in detox is by using a bentonite clay mask. The bentonite clay is amazing at supporting detox, is fairly inexpensive, and very easy to use. You'll add a scoop of the bentonite clay and water (follow the package for exact amounts) and once you have your paste, you apply it to your armpits. Allow to dry until it is light in color and wash off. Consider prioritizing activities that make you sweat to support your beautiful innately intelligent body.

Another way to support your body odor is to be mindful of your toxic load. A toxic load is how much exposure you have to toxins. This can be through feminine products as discussed in an earlier chapter, personal care products, cleaning products, water, food, air, lawn care, air fresheners, candles, etc. The three areas where toxins have the biggest impact on your health are food, cleaning, and personal care. The goal with looking at ingredients and being aware of your toxic load is not to eliminate 100% of your toxin exposure. This is simply not realistic and could drive you nuts. The goal, instead, is to lessen the burden of exposure on your body. God, in His infinite wisdom, created your body to process and detoxify poisons and toxins that can cause harm to your body. The problem comes when our body can't keep up with the detoxification process.

It's like a bucket with a small hole in the bottom. When you first start to slowly fill the bucket with water, it can more easily empty through the hole. But when the bucket starts to get full or the water going in increases in speed, you end up with a bucket that is overflowing. The little hole in the bottom can't keep up with emptying. This is the idea with your body's detox organs such as the liver. It has amazing pathways to eliminate harmful things, but when there's too much, it can't keep up with detoxing your body.

I'm going to keep my recommendations about which ingredients/toxins to avoid somewhat vague because these lists keep changing. For example, parabens and phthalates were placed on the hot seat and now most personal care products on the shelves tote being paraben and phthalate free. However, labeling can get away with tricks because companies can use "fragrance" which includes toxic ingredients such as parabens and phthalates. Just because the product doesn't have a specific ingredient doesn't mean it isn't hidden in another—like the term "fragrance" which can be thousands of toxins in just "one" listed ingredient.

In general, the best rule of thumb when looking at ingredients in any and all products is to look for ingredients you can pronounce and look for products with the fewest ingredients. You can ask the question: did God make it? Or did man make it? Lean toward what God made. It can be very overwhelming if you are new to reading labels. When I first started looking at ingredients, I researched them first and then kept a list in my phone so when I went to the store I had a reference or cheat sheet. One decent starting point for ingredients is the Environmental Working Group's website, EWG.org. This is where I gained my confidence in reading labels and from there I started to trust my own intuition and grow.

Food
Eat with nature. Health trends can be so confusing. Today we're only eating a carnivore diet, tomorrow only a plant-based diet is best. We're avoiding all carbs, no we're avoiding all fat, no it's the

sugar, no it's the salt! The pendulum keeps swinging from one extreme to another. It's enough to make your head spin.

A faith-based diet is simply: eat real food that God created for you to eat. There was a meme floating around social media of a depiction of an angel talking to God saying, "The people are making milk out of almonds."

God replies, "What?! But I gave them like eight animals they could get milk from."

This made me chuckle the first time I saw it, but beyond the joke in it, it has some truth to it. God gave us everything we need to survive, why are we complicating it and taking it into our own hands (or labs)? I've also heard a saying to help you think about this concept that goes, "If it comes from a plant—eat it. If it's made in a plant—don't eat it." Eating real, whole foods (from plants and animals) will always be healthier for you than something that has been processed and fortified with artificial food-like substances.

God made so many wonderful foods for us to eat. When you are considering the food you eat, be intentional with your ingredients. Ideally you want fresh, real, whole ingredients as the bulk of your diet. The fewer chemicals used in the production of your food, the better. Why do these things matter? Because there are so many food additives and chemicals used that interfere with our hormones. Everything in your body is connected, so if you are having digestive issues, your hormones and cycle will also be affected. Keeping all of your systems working properly keeps your hormones happy, too.

Don't forget to eat with God, too. Praying before meals, thanking the cook, thanking the animals or the earth for giving you your meal, all of these practices are extremely beneficial for your health. I made a meal for dinner that I had made a thousand times before, but that night the meal was particularly delicious. I made a comment to my family that it was exceptionally yummy, they agreed, and then my daughter said she knew why it tasted better that night—it was because she and her brother weren't fighting, I was calm, and enjoying my time in the kitchen putting lots of love into the food.

I told her I thought she was on to something there. Not just because I wanted to encourage them to not be wild and crazy while I was trying to cook, but because there's actually evidence that the more calm, love, and gratitude you put into your meal, the better your food will taste and serve you. When I was in school to get my certification in health coaching, one of the lecturers discussed a study where people were given slices of oranges. The ones that people gave thanks to were deemed tastier than the ones that weren't given thanks.

Now, I'm sure you're thinking what I thought the first time I heard this study—it doesn't seem legit.

Then I started learning more about Dr. Masaru Emoto's work with water and how water molecules change based on the emotions, thoughts, and environment it is in. He looked at the molecules of water after interacting with positive intentions and after interacting with negative intentions. The imagery shows solid structures in the water with positive intentions and a blurred molecular structure with negative intentions.

63

Between both works of thanking food and water, I started thinking about how maybe it's the water in the food that is creating molecular structures from the positivity making food taste better.

Whether you believe and trust these studies or not, it's hard to deny it entirely. Have you ever eaten something that your mom or someone you really love made for you and no matter how many times you cook the exact same recipe it just never tastes quite right? It's hard to deny the logic that our emotions affect the food we are eating or at least how we are experiencing the food.

Cleaning

Clean with nature. When you are cleaning, consider using products that don't disturb your thyroid. Bleach/chlorine decimates your thyroid function which is hugely instrumental in your endocrine (hormone) system. I used to use the cleaners that were bleach-based and would always feel like my lungs were on fire afterward. Every single cleaner in your home can be swapped out for equal parts water and vinegar with some essential oils. It's all I use to clean my home and I don't have to worry about damaging my thyroid or breaking the bank. This cleaner is cheap and easy to make.

Personal Care

Take care of yourself with nature. When you are thinking about personal care products such as cleansers, lotions, or make-up, consider looking for products that don't use parabens, phthalates, sodium lauryl sulfates, aluminum, petroleum-based ingredients, PEGs or fragrance. Again, these ingredients are endocrine disruptors and can cause chaos to your hormones. Just like food, look for ingredients that are real. If you wouldn't ingest it, why would you rub it into your body's largest organ to be absorbed into your bloodstream?

Fasting

Sacrificing animals to God was a common practice until the ultimate lamb was sacrificed—Jesus Christ. Then we see Jesus encourage people to fast in Matthew 6:16-18 (NIV) when he says, "When you fast, do not look somber as the hypocrites do, for they disfigure their faces to show others they are fasting. Truly I tell you, they have received their reward in full. But when you fast, put oil on your head and wash your face, so that it will not be obvious to others that you are fasting, but only to your Father, who is unseen; and your Father, who sees what is done in secret, will reward you." Instead of encouraging them to burn the fat of animals (how they sacrificed animals for God) to gain God's favor, He encouraged His followers to fast in private for the Lord. Fasting is also a way to burn fat in your body. When you are fasting, as a woman, it is going to be different than as a man. Our bodies are different no matter how hard other people try to convince us otherwise. The best time for your female body to fast is during your follicular phase right after your bleeding stops. During this phase, as you read earlier, your estrogen is rising and your body needs support in detoxing those extra hormones which fasting can also support. This is the phase in which your appetite is generally suppressed as well, so intermittent fasting is better tolerated. Intermittent fasting can be done by choosing a window of time each day you don't eat (called fasting). Many people do a 16/8 method meaning they fast for 16 hours and eat within a window of 8 hours. This amount is up to you and you can always change it. Be sure to stay properly hydrated always, but especially during fasting. Water with some Celtic sea salt for electrolytes is wonderful. Since this is not a medical advice book, always talk to your health care team and ultimately pray before you begin.

Lunaception and Moon Energy

There's a really cool phenomenon called *Lunaception* that many women use as a way to track, predict, and regulate their cycles.

Before doing health coach training, I was a public school teacher. The week of every full moon, I would hear my colleagues talk about how crazy the students were acting and blamed it on the impending full moon. I would roll my eyes at the thought that the full moon made students act any differently because, well, they were high energy every day…However, I started digging deeper into lunaception and lunar tracking; when I started to get intimately in tune with my own body, I started to realize and experience the power of the moon.

If you're like I once was and totally rolling your eyes at me right now, please hear me out. And if by the end of my soap box, you're still not into it, that's okay. Not everything is for everyone.

What is the first thing that comes to your mind when you're asked: what does the moon control? Do you think of tides? The power of the moon is so strong that it controls the tide in the ocean. It controls large bodies of water. Human bodies are on average 60% water, so we are also bodies of water that are controlled by the moon. As we get closer to nature, the more aligned we are with our bodies and purpose in life. In the creation story in Genesis 1:14 (NIV) "God says, 'Let there be lights in the vault of the sky to separate the day from the night, and let them serve as signs to mark sacred times, and days and years.'" Your period is an extremely sacred time in your life. Let the moon mark those sacred times as it is intended in Genesis 1.

Psalm 104:19 (NIV) says, "He made the moon to mark the

seasons, and the sun knows when to go down." The moon is so powerful and marks the seasons of your life as well as the seasons of nature. When women are living together, their cycles start to sync together. This is common and often joked about in entertainment. A father who has a wife and daughters often jokes (nervously) about them all syncing together and surviving the week. Not only do women sync together, but they also sync with the moon.

The seasons, the moon, menstruation…they're all cycles and they all sync together. We are nature and when we acknowledge that we are nature and start living more in alignment with it, we will start to see so much of our health mirrored in it.

Let's look closer at the moon.

I'm sure we've all gotten the same lesson about the phases of the moon. Maybe you were one of the lucky ones who got to use cookies and frosting to show each phase, maybe you colored them, or maybe you were just told to memorize the phases from a textbook. However you learned about the phases, you know the lesson I'm talking about.

Women who live very close to nature have cycles that sync with the moon with their ovulation during the full moon (when energy is high) and their periods with the new moon (when energy is low). Even the energies during the cycle mimic the moon's energies. However, modern day conveniences have disrupted our connection with nature causing us to have more of a separation from nature. We have artificial lighting inside and outside our homes and therefore spend more time indoors which disrupts our exposure to sun and moon light.

Wherever you are in your cycle, you can easily keep track of how you correspond to the moon by keeping track of when you get your period and what the moon is doing during that time. If you're not great at looking at the moon and knowing what phase it's in, you can search online for what the phase is in the night you get your period. If you are getting your period around the new moon, then you are probably ovulating around the full moon. Just as you are an observer using other tracking methods, looking at moon phases is no different. Don't fret if you are not ovulating during the full moon and bleeding during the new moon. Your cycle may not be exactly 28 days so your timing with the moon will rotate. As with everything in life, give yourself grace, acknowledge it, and live your life the way God intended you to. The closer you are to God, to the nature He created, to the purpose He has for your life—the better health you will experience.

Menopause and the Moon

There are so many cool things about the moon. If you are menopausal and want to still support your body using cycle syncing, you can use the phases of the moon. During the full moon you can support your body as though it is ovulating, during the waning moon you can support your body as though it's in the luteal phase, your period during the new moon, and your follicular phase during the waxing moon.

Irregularity, Amenorrhea, and Lunaception

Amenorrhea is when you are experiencing a time without a period that is not menopause. It's an abnormal pause in your period. An irregular period will vary for each woman. Generally speaking, cycles are anywhere between 24-38 days. You know your body best, so if you are having cycles about the same length each month, this is your regular.

Whether you are experiencing irregular periods or missing periods altogether, the moon has the power to regulate your cycles or get them kick started. This is called Lunaception. Here's what you do. Pay close attention and don't skip any steps.

1. Sleep with your curtains and/or windows open the night before the full moon, the night of the full moon, and the night after the full moon.
2. Sleep in complete darkness every other night.
3. Do this every month until your period comes back or gets regulated.

OR another method which works well if you live in a higher light polluted area:

1. Go outside every night for 5-10 minutes.
2. Look at the moon the entire time.
3. Go back to what you were doing when your time is up.

I know, I know, tricky, right? But that's how powerful the moon is! Just being or "bathing" in the moonlight can start up a lost period or regulate one that has gotten off course. God is so good and gave us all the tools we need for our health.

I can tell you firsthand that this works. I, again, was a huge skeptic, but thought I'd give it a shot. What was there to lose? So I slept with my curtains open for three nights during the full moon for a few months and my irregular period was regulated! Before you totally write it off as crazy, give it a shot. God gave us the moon and everything in nature. It's the most powerful form of health we have.

Testing and Bio-hacking

It's easy to let the noise of the world in. It takes over and tells you lies: how to look, feel, think, act, live. Unless the noise is rooted in faith, it's just noise and you don't have to give energy to it. You do not have to listen to or follow the crowd.

The newest tests or the newest "biohacking" gadgets designed in the name of health are also just noise. There have been a lot of trends in the health field. Buy this gadget, buy this product, buy this program. Buy. Buy. Buy. You do not have to spend a fortune to be healthy. In fact, the more artificial and away from nature you get, the less you will experience health.

God never intended for you to carry the weight of the world on your shoulders. His intention was not for you to be consumed by all the tragedies across the map. Have you heard the story of The Tower of Babel? It comes from Genesis 11:1-9 (NIV) and goes like this, "Now the whole world had one language and a common speech. As people moved eastward, they found a plain in Shinar and settled there. They said to each other, 'Come, let's make bricks and bake them thoroughly.' They used brick instead of stone, and tar for mortar. Then they said, 'Come, let us build ourselves a city, with a tower that reaches to the heavens, so that we may make a name for ourselves; otherwise we will be scattered over the face of the whole earth.' But the Lord came down to see the city and the tower the people were building. The Lord said, 'If as one people speaking the same language they have begun to do this, then nothing they plan to do will be impossible for them. Come, let us go down and confuse their language so they will not understand each other.' So the Lord scattered them from there over all the earth, and they stopped building the city. That is why it is called Babel—because there the Lord confused the language of the whole world. From there the Lord scattered them over the face of the whole earth."

In this story, it was very easy for the world to communicate because everyone spoke the same language. Whether or not people actually listened to one another is a different story altogether, but they did not have a language barrier. The people wanted to build their own city with a tower to reach the heavens. The people were deliberately disobeying God to build this tower and as a consequence, God scattered them and made it so everyone spoke a different language causing confusion and disharmony. If God had placed importance on His people being able to speak clearly to each other and to have the knowledge of the world, He would have found another consequence for the world.

It doesn't feel moral, but the problems of the world are not yours. Turn off your TV. Turn off the news. Turn off social media. Turn off the world. That does not make you an irresponsible citizen. It makes you a responsible daughter of Christ. There will always be problems in the world—and God will ALWAYS be the one who has control.

I'm not saying you should be naive to what's happening around you. Go out and talk with friends, family, neighbors. You don't have to live life with blinders on, but you don't have to let the problems of the world become yours either. Often the greatest impact you can have is within an arm's reach.

Just as God never intended for you to be consumed by the problems of the world, He also never intended for you to be in a constant update of the intricacies of your body. Society has become test crazed. So much so that it's no longer enough to go into a provider and get a test once a year. Many people are being tested 24/7/365. There are many tests you can take that can tell you information about your health. You can test for levels of hormones, vitamins/minerals, proper sleep, function of organs, food sensitivities/intolerances/allergies, etc. These are all options for you, of course, but I'm a firm believer that we are a society of over testers (and over spenders). I have noticed this influx of people (especially women) who are in a constant state of testing themselves. There are apps on phones and watches, rings, continuous glucose monitors for non-diabetics, even bed technologies that continuously monitor everything from breathing, heart rate, amount of sleep, and number of steps to fertility, hormone levels, and blood glucose. Your body's levels ebb and flow. That's what it's designed to do. There are conditions in which knowing some of this information is helpful, but these cases are not who I am speaking of. These numbers are being abused and the whole woman is being overlooked.

Remember, true foundational health is not just found on your plate—it's found in your lifestyle. Just as true health is not found in a number. All of a sudden health becomes a number; not a feeling, state of mind, state of being, or lifestyle. It often starts as an observation, but the stress of changing numbers, and controlling the numbers, takes hold of you and (very sneakily) you find yourself worrying more about a number on a test than you do about enjoying and living your full life.

Beyond the detriment of becoming number-focused instead of health-focused, another consequence of using these devices is that most of them (if not all of them) expose your body to EMF (electromagnetic field) which is manmade radiation and can really interfere with hormonal rhythms. This radiation is not the same as the radiation you receive from the sun—that's natural radiation which is beneficial for you. EMF exposure comes from things like cell phones, air pods, smart watches, any bluetooth technology, smart meters on your home, wireless internet, smart tvs, microwaves, and computers to name a few.

Another caution with testing is that I often hear women complain that something is not right—they don't feel well and they are following their intuition that something is off—but the doctor says nothing is wrong with them. They run all the blood panels and results come back normal. This is a very common story. And it's because there is so much more to health than what can be tested in a blood panel and most doctors aren't trained in holistic health. When done intentionally, testing can be a profound tool, but it has really gotten out of control.

Faith-based health is about getting back in touch with what's real. It's about getting back to nature. It's about getting back to God.

Mitigating Stress

I was streaming music while writing this book and an ad came on for online therapy. The ad began by saying that we don't come with an owner's manual and goes on to say there's nothing that tells us how to handle relationship issues or personal problems. Every time I heard this ad, I yelled out, "Yes we do! It's called the Bible." While the Bible isn't going to tell you specifics involving the intricacies of your unique life, it does have all the answers through story. The Bible has all the answers to relationships, health, menstruation, morality, life. However, when you drift away from it, you start to doubt the Word and trust God's plan less. Messages from the world are heavy that the Bible doesn't have the answers and to rely on other people. This disconnect from faith creates fear and stress which is the underlying cause of most health issues, especially menstrual issues. Open your Bible and see for yourself.

Modern science shows that stress can throw a woman's cycle off balance in a myriad of ways. Because stress triggers the release of cortisol, you see an interference in the hypothalamic-pituitary-gonadal (HPG) axis that regulates reproductive hormones such as estrogen and progesterone. Everything in your body is connected and it's no different for your hormones. Your hypothalamus and pituitary glands are located in your brain and send signals to many of your other organs and hormone-producing glands. When your hypothalamus and pituitary glands are disrupted it can disrupt more than just your reproductive hormones, which is why managing stress is important even if you are not experiencing issues with your cycle.

High levels of cortisol can also suppress gonadotropin-releasing hormone (GnRH) which can lead to irregular ovulation or missed periods (amenorrhea). When your body is releasing an egg delayed or not at all, your body will experience irregular or completely skipped cycles. Irregular and skipped cycles are very common amongst women in high-stress situations such as intense work schedules, emotional stress, or major life changes.

Stress can also lead to heavier or lighter bleeding than usual, more severe PMS, and more painful periods. Because stress affects the uterine lining, you can experience heavier periods (menorrhagia) and because it can also reduce estrogen and progesterone, you can experience lighter bleeding (hypomenorrhea). This is another reason why it is so important to observe your body and really get in tune with yourself because you are the one who determines these shifts from your "normal." PMS has become such a common occurrence with periods that no one really bats an eye to it anymore. Did you know that major mood swings, fatigue (extreme tiredness to the point of barely being able to function), cramping, major bloating, and head-aches are actually all signs that you're experiencing imbalances in your hormones or other levels of vitamins or minerals? Stress can exacerbate PMS by increasing inflammation and altering serotonin (happy hormone) levels which leads to unpleasant and sometimes life-disrupting symptoms associated with periods.

Since stress affects your body in such profound ways, it's really important to understand what it is, what causes you stress, how your body responds to stress, and what tools for managing stress work best for you.

There are two parts to your nervous system that are most asso-ciated with stress: sympathetic nervous system and parasym-pathetic nervous system. Your sympathetic nervous system is activated in times of stress and is often described as the "fight-or-flight" system. It prepares the body for stressful or emergency situations by increasing heart rate, dilating the pupils, and mobi-lizing energy. The parasympathetic nervous system is activated using the stress management tools in this book amongst other tools and is often described as the "rest and digest" system. It works to calm the body after stress, slowing the heart rate, and promoting digestion and relaxation. So even if you don't use any tools to manage stress, your body's parasympathetic nervous system will kick in—because your body is brilliantly designed. However, using these tools can help you recover from stress quicker.

Stressors come in all shapes and sizes. They can be physical, mental, and emotional and everyone experiences stress differently. It is perceived and manifested in as many ways as there are people on this earth. Your life experiences impact the way you perceive stress. Two people can experience the same event; one can perceive it as stressful and the other can be unphased. It's just like the saying—*one man's trash is another man's treasure.* We see the world around us based on who we are, not the way things are. We also have stressors that are physical and just as some people cope with emotional or mental stress differently, we also cope with physical stress uniquely. For instance, if I were to run a marathon right now my body would experience tremendous physical stress. (Okay, I'll be honest, even if I were to run a few miles I'd experience tremendous physical stress). However, for someone who trains and is prepared, running a marathon would not cause the same level of physical stress.

There are two main types of stress: short-term and long-term; also known as chronic stress. When I refer to stress that is damaging our health, I'm referring to chronic stress.

Everything we consume has the potential to stress us. Most people think about eating when thinking about the word consume, but we consume ideas, energies, thoughts, sights, sounds, feelings, vibes, etc. You can eat a perfect meal plan to support your body and hormones during each of your phases of your cycle, but if you are consuming fear, stress, anxiety, negativity, etc. it doesn't matter. I'm not saying eating well and being aware of the products you use doesn't matter. Those can also be physical stressors if your body isn't properly prepared to process them or if it is being overly exposed to them, but it's only one piece of the thousand piece puzzle.

Before I became a mom and my mom brain developed with heightened awareness of danger, I was really into Law and Order: SVU (Special Victims Unit), so it's about a lot of sex crimes and crimes against children. When I say it like that, I wonder why anyone would be interested in a show about that. Anyway, there was always a lot of suspense and it really got my mind and heart racing. That kind of suspense was driving my stress level WILD without me realizing it. You see, my brain knew that what I was seeing on TV was just TV and was not a true story. What I was seeing was based on a true story (as the show says in the intro), but the actual people I was seeing weren't real and the details weren't real either. My brain knew that. My body, though, didn't know that. My body was in fight, flight, freeze, fawn mode as a response to this stress. So it was preparing me to either need to fight, escape or run away, freeze and do nothing, or to please an adversary in order to save my own life. Again, I knew I was safe, but because my brain was perceiving this show as stressful and dangerous or scary, it was kicking my body into high gear.

This type of response is actually a good thing. You need your body to respond to stress because if there really is a dangerous situation, you need to activate your responses. However, you need to be very careful not to put undue stress on your body especially if you are already feeling high stress. It's important to be mindful of everything you consume throughout each day.

One of the sermons I recently heard at church was about saving the best for last. The preacher was talking about when Jesus was turning the water into wine at the wedding at Cana and how usually the customary/traditional practice was to serve your best wine first and then your lesser value wine later once everyone had their fill of wine, but what Jesus did when they ran out of wine was turned the water into a really amazing wine and the guests were commenting, "Wow! You saved the best for last!" This was a novelty and rare occurrence. This section on stress, yes, might be at the end of the chapter, but it is by far the best thing you can do for your overall health because pretty much any issue healthwise can be brought back to the impact that stress has on your body; which is why when I talk about any sort of a change that you could make to your lifestyle, I don't want you to stress about it. If you are making these changes and you're losing joy in going out and experiencing your life because you're too hyper-focused on what you're eating, or you're eating foods that you think are so disgusting—this mentality is working against you just as much as the toxins.

There are many band-aids that women use to mitigate their stress. And when it comes to short-term stress, these band-aids can absolutely absolve your stress. However, when it comes to chronic stress, you need solutions that truly make a difference in your stress level. For instance, taking a vacation or a break from your day-to-day grind can be helpful if you had an isolated stressful event and can use the break as a reset. A short-term way to cope with short-term stress. When you have chronic stress, though, the stress is still waiting for you when you get home. You'd be using your vacation to escape your life, and then after that little reprieve from your stress, you're just going right back to a life that causes you insurmountable stress.

Vacations are great, don't get me wrong. I love to travel, but they are not the solution to a stressful life. They're just a short-term solution to a long-term issue. But the stress that is harming your health is the chronic stress. The lifestyle stress. Your stressful life is still waiting for you when you get home so in order for you to truly address your stress, you really have to be looking at all of the aspects of your life and everything you consume, not just what's on your plate. You can eat the most meticulously planned-out meal plan for the rest of your life, but if you are constantly having to go to, let's say, a job that you absolutely hate—you pull up to that building every day and start having a visceral reaction to just being in that place, this stress will do more damage than your uber healthy meals will do good.

If there's only one piece of advice you take away from this book, I hope that it is to identify and mitigate chronic stress.

One of the biggest issues that impacts our hormones is stress. If any of the recommendations in this book cause you to feel stressed out or anxious, please don't follow them and give yourself some grace. There is nothing about health and wellness that is worth it if it causes you to stress out.

Just as the Bible tells us many times that we should rest, it is very abundant in reference to fear. When you boil down stress and anxiety, what you find is fear. Fear is the base or the root of stress and anxiety. And God is very clear in the Bible about fear and how we should treat it. He point-blank tells us to not be afraid. The Bible is filled with the same message: do not fear. This aligns with God's call for trust in Him in the Bible. Psalm 46:10 (NIV) is a beautiful reminder to trust in God's promise that he is in control of all circumstances when it says, "Be still and know that I am God; I will be exalted among the nations, I will be exalted in the earth." When we trust in Him and surrender our stress to Him, our bodies function the way He intended.

Growing up, I was a part of the children's choir at church and my favorite song, a song that has stuck with me my whole life, was "You Are Mine." It is based on the verse from the Bible from Isaiah 43:1-7 (NIV) that says, "...Do not fear, for I have redeemed you; I have summoned you by name; you are mine. When you pass through the waters, I will be with you; and when you pass through the rivers, they will not sweep over you. When you walk through the fire, you will not be burned; the flames will not set you ablaze. For I am the Lord your God, the Holy One of Israel, your Savior; I give Egypt for your ransom, Cush and Seba in your stead. Since you are precious and honored in my sight, and because I love you, I will give people in exchange for you, nations in exchange for your life. Do not be afraid, for I am with you; I will bring your children from the east and gather you from the west. I will say to the north, 'Give them up!' and to the south, 'Do not hold them back.' Bring my sons from afar and my daughters from the ends of the earth—everyone who is called by my name, whom I created for my glory, whom I formed and made." Do not be afraid, God is with you! What a beautiful message. God is so good.

2 Timothy 1:7 is a great reminder of how God created us. "For the Spirit God gave us does not make us timid, but gives us power, love, and self-discipline." Wow. What an empowering message. You may experience fear, stress, anxiety, but it is not by the design of your spirit. You have a powerful, loving, and self-disciplined spirit. You are not broken, there is nothing wrong with you. You are so wonderfully made. The things causing you stress are challenges that your powerful spirit can overcome. God has a great plan for you.

When I think of Psalm 34:4 (NIV) - "I sought the Lord, and he answered me; he delivered me from all my fears," I think, *All you have to do is ask.* Seek out God, seek out an intimate relationship with Jesus, seek out power in your faith, and you will be reprieved of your fears.

Proverbs 29:25 (NIV) says, "Fear of man will prove to be a snare, but whoever trusts in the Lord is kept safe." Fear is, unfortunately, a widely used tactic of controlling the masses because, as the Bible says, fear is a snare. The lies, the hyperbole, the threats—they're all carefully designed to induce fear and cause anxiety; stress out the system and create compliance to someone or something other than God. Our Lord and savior is more powerful than all of that chaos as long as you trust in Him, you are safe. You do not have to listen to the fear spread about because you know who your true savior is.

So how is it possible that you as a woman of faith could still experience stress and anxiety? Well, it's a lot easier said than done, right? It takes practice to give over all of your fears to God and to fully trust in His plan.

We are bombarded daily with words, images, messages, and thoughts that are skillfully crafted to keep us in a state of fear. They're not real; they're all lies. But we believe them. We take them in and accept them as truth. We are human and God knows this. He's there waiting for you to return to Him and give Him your struggles. He WANTS you to give Him your pain, suffering, trials and tribulations, and fear.

When it comes to your menstruation, you can really start to see the parallel between how your body responds to stress and any discrepancies you might observe in your menstrual cycle. When you stress out, your menstruation can be affected in a number of ways: it can stop (amenorrhea), it can become irregular, it can increase symptoms of **PMS** (mood swings, cramps, acne), among other complications and disruptions. It's not uncommon for women who are avid runners to experience amenorrhea due to the physical stress placed on their bodies. It's not uncommon for women who experience great loss to also experience amenorrhea due to the emotional and mental stress.

Beyond effects to your menstruation, your body can experience a myriad of negative impacts from stress such as: a higher risk of heart disease, heart attack, stroke, high blood pressure, weakened intestinal barrier, sleep disorders like insomnia, weight gain, muscle tension, pain, headaches, anxiety, depression, memory loss, brain fog, and so much more. Like I have said a few times already—stress is the root of health issues.

It can be daunting looking at the number of potential stressors in your life and how to manage them. There isn't a perfect test you can take to get a clear answer on what is stressing you out due to the fact that your perception of stress is different from another person's perception and strategies you already have implemented in your life to manage your stress. My hope is that the information shared here will serve as a tool kit for you to be able to observe and identify stressors in your life and what strategies work best for you to manage them.

Sleep
Stress has a huge impact on sleep just as it impacts your menstrual cycle. Sleep is incredibly important for your body in a million ways. Sleep is life-changing and if it hasn't been made

clear yet, REST is key to health. Have you ever woken up from a full night's sleep and felt like a million bucks? What about the opposite: wake up feeling like you were hit by a bus, still tired, and feeling like you have to be pulled out of bed? Now ask yourself how often you feel like a million bucks vs how many you wake feeling unrested. If you're feeling unrested more than rested, looking at your sleep hygiene and what is affecting your sleep is an important step in your health journey.

Your body does a lot of work in the shadows of the night to keep you functioning properly. This is a nutshell version of how stress impacts sleep. It's important for your body to process and get rid of toxic waste which happens when you sleep. When you don't get quality sleep, the toxic waste builds up in your brain and nervous system which is why you wake up with clouded thoughts and moody emotions.

Your amygdala, which is located in the temporal lobe in your brain, controls your reaction when you face a perceived threat or stress. When you get enough quality sleep, your amygdala can react in a more adaptive way because it's not overburdened with excess toxins or emotions, which is why when you are sleep deprived, you experience heightened emotions and can overreact.

Sleep and stress create a vicious cycle. When you are stressed out, you lose sleep. And when you are short on sleep, you create stress in your body. But fear not, because there are tools you can use to get better sleep.

Getting to bed at a decent/early time isn't always easy though, and it's not always because you aren't tired and ready to sleep.

There are many common obstacles or challenges to getting to sleep at an earlier time.

- Screen time and blue light:
  - ° Your screens—TV, computer, cell phones, LED lights, etc. emit blue light which disrupts your body's natural ability to produce melatonin (the hormone that helps you get sleepy). One way to support better sleep is to shut off your screen devices about two hours before going to bed. This way your body can recover from all of the blue light from the day better and start the production of melatonin.
- Overstimulation:
  - ° When you engage in intense conversations, participate in an exciting activity, or scroll your night away on social media (which is also exposing you to blue light) right before bed, you are keeping your brain wired. Just as you can turn off blue light emitting technologies two hours before bed, you can also choose to not participate in these over-stimulating activities before bed. Sometimes, this is unavoidable, right? There's a concert, event, or something on TV that you really want to see. Sometimes you have social and work commitments that keep you out late, but you have the power to create habits of lessening stimulation before bed to form a restful bedtime routine.
- Inconsistent routine and lack of wind-down time:
  - ° Routine is so incredibly important when it comes to health. Your habits create your health more than anything else. In regards to sleep, routine would look like going to bed and waking up at a consistent time.

Having a special wind down routine that you can do consistently is also important to support proper rest. This routine is something that signals to your body that it's time for rest. Your wind-down routine could look something like this: brush teeth, wash face, change into pajamas, pray, lie down. It does not have to be something extravagant.

- Caffeine and late-night eating:
  - Drinking caffeinated beverages can affect people in different ways, but the bottom line is that caffeine is a stimulant and can interfere with sleep. Along with that is eating late at night. When you eat too close to bedtime, your body is focusing on digesting what you just ate instead of focusing on resting.
- Stress and anxiety:
  - It's hard to fall asleep when you have a racing mind worried about all the realistic and unrealistic what-ifs in life. A great practice to get into is praying. Give it to God! (And go to sleep).
- Environmental factors:
  - Your bedroom environment is an important piece of getting to sleep. If you have too much noise (overstimulating your brain even in sleep), too much light, an uncomfortable mattress or pillow, or if it's too hot or too cold can all affect your ability to fall asleep.
- Second wind effect:
  - Have you ever felt tired and then once you have a chance to go to bed, you get a burst of energy? If only this second wind came mid-afternoon! This energy boost when you're trying to go to bed is the antithesis to what is conducive to falling asleep.

- Time management:
  - ° You are a busy person and the end of the day is often time to get everything done that you weren't able to do during the day. This is often when you get to spend time with a spouse or significant other, time to decompress and have some time with the Word, or time to work on a hobby you love. It's easy to lose track of time and unintentionally get to bed later than intended.

Earlier I talked about the vicious cycle of not getting enough sleep causing stress and stress causing you to not get enough sleep. This cycle is why creating a calming bedtime routine is so crucial for your health. Because reducing stress is one way to get quality sleep (and getting quality sleep in turn lessens your stress). See? This cycle can actually work in your favor!

Now, I could share with you my bedtime routine and you could copy my routine, but what works for me might not work for you. Without knowing you and your lifestyle, I can't say you should just do xyz and you will get perfect quality sleep! I wish it was that easy. However, there are general guidelines to creating an optimal bedtime routine such as:

-starting a winding down process an hour before you plan to fall asleep
-go to bed at a consistent time every night (or at least the majority of nights)
-put away all electronics or any screen emitting blue light at least an hour before bed
-limit your EMF exposure by turning off WiFi at night, keeping your cell phone away from your bed or at least turning it to airplane mode

-create a comfortable and cozy environment for yourself
-do a calming activity

Again, I can't tell you exactly how your routine should look or the activities that you should do to calm yourself down. These are very individualized habits that you would form to create your own routine. This is simply a list of ideas to help you brainstorm your own routine.

Dance

Dancing, whether done in public or in the confines of your home with no one to witness, is an exceptionally overlooked and underrated stress reliever. It's a form of movement that triggers the release of endorphins, the body's natural "feel good" hormones, which help reduce stress and improve mood. While the endorphins are rising, your cortisol levels are lowering. Studies show that dancing can lower cortisol, the hormone associated with stress, helping to create a sense of calm. Focusing on movement and rhythm (even if you're way off beat dancing to the beat of your own drum) can help bring awareness to the present moment, similar to meditation, reducing anxious thoughts.

Have you ever gotten to a point where there are so many stressors trying to create chaos in your life and you have no idea what your true feelings really are or how to express them with words? Dance can help. It allows you to express emotions nonverbally so you can release pent up tension and process feelings in a healthy way. You can dance in any way you desire to whatever music you enjoy. If the thought of dancing makes you uncomfortable, start with a gentle hip sway side to side. It doesn't have to be well done choreography. It doesn't even have to really be what you might define as dancing. What's really happening when you are dancing is called somatic movement which includes movements such as clapping, stomping, swaying, shaking, pumping, jumping, etc. Somatic movement supports your body in moving the energy that is otherwise stuck in your body creating stress.

In case you need more encouragement to dance, the Bible makes reference to dancing in both testaments and in times of celebration, worship, and sorrow as well. In the Old Testament, in Exodus 15:20-21, Miriam, the prophetess, led the women in dancing and singing after the Israelites followed Moses across the Red Sea to escape Egypt. In an earlier chapter you read about King David in 2 Samuel 6:14-16 when King David was dancing with all his might before the Ark of the Covenant throughout the streets. Celebrate your life with dance. Wake up in the morning and celebrate that God gave you another day!

Psalm 149:3 (NIV) says, "Let them praise his name with dancing and make music to him with timbrel and harp," and basically saying the same thing, Psalm 150:4 (NIV) says, "Praise him with timbrel and dancing, praise him with the strings and pipe," so if you are looking for a better reason to dance than stress relief or celebration, do it to praise God.

In Ecclesiastes 3:4 (NIV), there is a well-known verse: "A time to weep and a time to laugh, a time to mourn and a time to dance." Trust in God's timing and know that the highs and the lows are all a part of the human experience. The use of dance is to show a time of celebration, but what if we also used dance in times of stress, sorrow, or grief? It's predominantly seen as an expression of celebration, but it can be a profound tool for healing in times when celebration feels far away.

Luke 15:11-32 (NIV) is a story about a son who squandered his inheritance and abandoned his family for many years. He spent all of his money, had no means to live where he was, and ran back home with his tail between his legs saying, "Father, I have sinned against heaven and against you. I am no longer worthy to be called your son." Instead of casting his son away for hurting him so deeply, the father welcomed him in and threw a celebration with dancing. The older son who stayed with their father was mad about the feast, but the father explained his compassion and forgiveness for the prodigal son. Even when life expectations fall short and people hurt you, finding forgiveness and dancing to celebrate your forgiveness can be such a monumental way to heal. Remember, forgiveness is for you—not them. To forgive someone, even if they don't ask for forgiveness, frees you from the prison of anger, stress, and chaos.

Gratitude

It's really easy to be grateful when life is going your way. Something good happens and it's all, "Thank you, God!" and when something bad happens it's all, "WHY GOD?!?!" I get it. I do it too. But when you lead with a grateful heart you are better guarding yourself against stress. One strategy to cultivate more gratitude in your life is to create a journal that is for listing what you're grateful for. Pick a time every day that you will write three things in your journal that you are grateful for from the last time you wrote in your gratitude journal. It's okay if you repeat. Some days you will notice that this task is very easy and you may have more than three things you're grateful for. Other days you will struggle with this because not all days are rainbows and butterflies. This is okay. You're living the human experience and you are not given the same circumstances day in and day out. 1 Thessalonians 5:18 says, "Give thanks in all circumstances; for this is God's will for you in Christ Jesus." God wants us to have a grateful heart. This is not the same as "toxic positivity." You can still be upset about a situation and be grateful. These two things are not just isolated feelings just as feeling joy in your life during dark times can be synonymous.

Journaling

Journaling also has a profound impact on stress. A journal, or diary, is a safe space for you to pour your heart out without judgment. You can do this as a part of your routine or use it when you are really feeling like you need to vent your issues, but consistency gives best results when using journaling as a stress managing tool. Journaling can help you process your emotions and prevent them from becoming overwhelming while organizing your thoughts and gaining insights into your stressors. It can help you to see your situations from a new perspective as well when you reread what you have written. When you look back on previous journal entries, you have the ability to notice any patterns in your stress and brainstorm solutions to those for your future. Writing in a journal keeps you present and mindful in a situation and can keep you from being overwhelmed by anxious thoughts. Instead of suppressing your worries, you can write them on the pages of a journal to reduce overthinking the situation. Don't worry if you're not a writer. You can always do a voice to text on your computer, phone, or other device. Package away your mental clutter and try journaling.

Primary Foods

One way to navigate lessening your stress is to look at primary foods. When it comes to food, there are primary foods and secondary foods. You might be surprised, but the food on your plate is actually secondary food. In the Bible in Matthew 4:4 (NIV), it says, "Jesus answered, 'It is written, "Man shall not live on bread alone, but on every word that comes from the mouth of God.""" Bread or food is not what we are to live solely on. There is more to our health than just the food we eat. We are not meant to live on 'bread alone.' The primary foods that have the largest impacts on your life are: Creativity, Finances, Career, Education, Health, Physical Activity, Home Cooking, Home Environment, Relationships, Social Life, Joy, and Spirituality. Each of these primary foods feeds your body and nourishes your soul in different ways contributing to your health outcomes.

Creativity is not just about being an artist. It even goes beyond being crafty. There is creativity in putting outfits together, organizing a closet, or solving a problem. Isaiah 64:8 (NIV) says, "Yet you, Lord, are our Father. We are the clay, you are the potter; we are all the work of your hand," which reminds us that God is our ultimate creator. He is always shaping and molding our lives just as we are experiencing the creativity of shaping and molding our lives through Him.

Finance is a pretty straightforward area. How are you with the money you have and what are your beliefs about the money you want to have? This is also where beliefs and feelings of abundance come in. Is abundance defined solely on the number you see in your bank account or is there more to abundance than that? Hebrews 13:5 (NIV) says, "Keep your lives free from the love of money and be content with what you have, because God has said, 'Never will I leave you; never will I forsake you.'" This can be a very tricky primary food because it is often where people find most issues with trusting God. You need money to live; that's just the reality of it. This is not to suggest that everyone should just quit working or making a living, but this is to serve as a challenge to really gauge how deeply you trust in God's plan for you.

Career is how you feel about what you do. This could be a job you get paid for or the life work you wake up to every day. Do you feel like you are living God's purpose? Proverbs 16:3 (NIV) says, "Commit to the Lord whatever you do, and he will establish your plans." Beyond thinking about your purpose, which has a gigantic impact on our overall health, is asking: is what you're doing as a career aligning with what God wants out of you? It makes me think of the saying that's very popular that comes from Matthew 19:26 that says, "through Him all things are possible." Yes, the impossible is possible with God, but it has to be God's will for you. As we see in countless stories in the Bible, especially with figures like King Saul in 1 Samuel, God will move mountains and help you overcome as long as you are following His call for your life. King Saul was anointed the first king over Israel by God Himself. Throughout Saul's kingship, you see that he makes decisions that go against God's will. This angers God and eventually leads to his removal from the throne of Israel. If you are doing God's will, he will make the impossible possible. So when you are considering your career, consider more than just how much money you earn or how much you enjoy it. Also consider God's purpose for you. Big life questions, but always good to keep in mind.

Education, for many, is viewed as a hurdle they leapt over to get to their adulthood, but education is the continuation of your learning. It goes far beyond formal education. This is lifelong learning. Do you feel like you are continuing to learn and grow? 2 Timothy 2:15 (NIV) says, "Do your best to present yourself to God as one approved, a worker who does not need to be ashamed and who correctly handles the word of truth." This verse is talking about your continued learning and seeking to learn the truth and decipher it from lies. Consider not just your continued learning of things of the flesh (things of the world around you) but also about your faith. What is your knowledge of God, Jesus, the Bible? I can tell you right now that you are excelling in this category just from the fact that when you heard about this book, you decided you wanted to learn more. You are leaps and bounds ahead of so many other women who haven't taken the initiative to learn more, so I can tell you already value your lifelong learning in growing closer to Christ.

There's a popular saying that many believe to stem from the Bible (but it's actually a Chinese proverb) that says, "Give a man a fish, he'll eat for a day. Teach a man to fish, he'll eat for life." Many believe that this stems from Jesus teaching people how to fish. And in itself, it is a great lesson that learning something for yourself is far more powerful than someone else doing it for you. However, in Matthew 4:19 (NIV), Jesus tells Simon and Andrew, "Come, follow me…and I will send you out to fish for people." This story goes beyond the Chinese proverb of fishing. What the Bible is really referring to is teaching others about the faith. The net that is cast out is not a net to gather fish, but is a metaphor for the teaching and sharing of faith you do in your life to further your education and the education of others around you. It means showing others how a life of faith is one of peace and love and to teach through being an example of that.

Health encompasses many aspects. How do you feel in general? Are you currently managing any chronic issues? How is your sleep? 1 Corinthians 6:19-20 (NIV) says, "Do you not know that your bodies are temples of the Holy Spirit, who is in you, whom

93

you have received from God? You are not your own; you were bought at a price. Therefore honor God with your bodies." Your body is a tool through which your soul should honor God. Jesus died for you. He paid the ultimate price for you to live. Paul wrote this letter to the Corinthians because he wanted to warn them about using their bodies for God's glory and not for the lustful desires of the flesh. When you think about your body in terms of being a temple, do you feel like you are honoring it in a holy way? If you don't think you are, I know that you at least want to, just by reading this book. You are taking steps to support and honor your temple. And that's a step in the right direction.

Physical activity is synonymous with movement. I don't like the word exercise. I think many people have negative connotations when it comes to "exercise" perhaps because images of gym class come to mind and using their period as an excuse to get out of it comes to play with the word. Therefore, when you think about your physical activity, I want you to consider your intentional movement. Do you take walks, go for jogs, or take a movement/ fitness class? It can also be the movement you naturally do in your day. Are you walking or riding your bike to work? It really boils down to how active or sedentary your lifestyle is and how you feel about it, not in a comparison way. Just because a woman you follow on social media works out daily, which is more than you do, doesn't mean you aren't satisfied with the amount of movement you get. Your health and satisfaction with your health is about you—and no one else.

1 Corinthians 9:24-27 (NIV) says, "Do you not know that in a race all the runners run, but only one gets the prize? Run in such a way as to get the prize. Everyone who competes in the games goes into strict training. They do it to get a crown that will not

last, but we do it to get a crown that will last forever. Therefore I do not run like someone running aimlessly; I do not fight like a boxer beating the air. No, I strike a blow to my body and make it my slave so that after I have preached to others, I myself will not be disqualified for the prize." If you know much about history or geography, Corinth was a Greek city state, so Paul was writing in a way that this Greek city state would understand. Think Greek Olympics here; people who value physical performance and active lifestyle. He's really using the race analogy to say they need to be just as self-disciplined in their physical goals as they are in their spiritual goals, but this can go both ways. We need to be physically and spiritually disciplined because as it was stated before—your body is your temple. And this message still stands today. Society places an emphasis of importance on physical appearance and activity. Weight loss programs, health programs, etc. all center around physical activity or exercise. This verse from the Bible is a great reminder of the self-discipline needed for a physical and spiritual life.

Home cooking alone can transform your health in a huge way. When you are making your own food, you are in control of the ingredients. Not everyone is a Michelin star chef, but you don't have to be. Start small if you're uncomfortable with home cooking. Make one meal. Start with "semi" homemade where you still use some pre-made ingredients and work your way to cooking from scratch. 1 Corinthians 10:31 (NIV) says, "So whether you eat or drink or whatever you do, do it all for the glory of God." When you are preparing meals in your home it is a way to grow closer in your relationship with God. You are providing nourishment for yourself, your family, friends, or the hungry. I have read and heard the most amazing connections between Jesus and bread making. When you make bread, you have to knead the dough. Kneading is the process where you are rough with the dough; you basically beat it up just as Jesus was beaten and ultimately crucified. After the kneading process, you let the dough rest just as Jesus was then laid to rest. The reason you let the dough rest is because that's when the dough RISES! JUST AS JESUS ROSE! Cue the chills. This story completely changed the way I think about bread making. Home cooking can be a way to connect to Jesus and your faith.

Home environment speaks to the physical and energetic aspects of your home. When you walk in your home, do you feel relaxed or tense? What is the level of organization in your home? A cluttered space creates a cluttered mind. Isaiah 32:18 (NIV) says, "My people will live in peaceful dwelling places, in secure homes, in undisturbed places of rest." Home is meant to be a place of rest, peace, and calm. Creating a space, even if it's not your entire home, just one space if that's what's available, that aids you in tranquility, can have a huge impact on your life.

Relationships greatly influence our overall health. God did not create us to be alone; hence he created Eve to be with Adam. We are social creatures by nature. What are your relationships like? This goes beyond just romantic relationships, too. Think about every person in your life. If you are in a relationship with someone who ushers chaos into your life, this relationship is not serving your health. 1 Corinthians 15:33 (NIV) says, "Do not be mislead: 'Bad company corrupts good character.'" It is okay to love someone and let them go. There's a saying, "Show me your friends and I'll show you your future," and it's so true. If you are consistently surrounding yourself with gossip and drama, you are furthering yourself from your relationship with God. Your relationship with God should be first and foremost as a woman of faith. This is the relationship that is the foundation for all other relationships.

Social life is another fairly obvious area of health. It is closely related to relationships, but more so speaks to the balance between work and play. How often do you see your friends in real life? Social media has had its benefits, but it simply does not replace human interaction. Hebrews 10:24-25 (NIV) says, "And let us consider how we may spur one another on toward love and good deeds, not giving up meeting together, as some are in the habit of doing, but encouraging one another—and all the more as you see the Day approaching." Gathering with others is crucial for our spirit and overall health. When we are united together, we are powerful. We share our ideas, we share our struggles, we share our triumphs. This is a vital piece of the human experience and of the faith.

Joy has to be the most underrated and overlooked area of health. God wants you to live a peaceful and joyful life, but this is often confused with a happy life. You can feel peace and joy in chaos. Joy is a state of mind even in the darkest of hours. Happiness is temporary and fleeting. Peace and joy are states of mind. Your level of joy in your life is easiest to assess during the hard times. Are you able to still see the light and thank God for the innumerable blessings He has bestowed upon your life even when the world seems like it's crumbling around you? That's joy. James 1:2-3 (NIV) says, "Consider it pure joy, my brothers and sisters, whenever you face trials of many kinds, because you know that the testing of your faith produces perseverance." I often see shirts and various other objects with the saying, "Count it All Joy!" It's a wonderful reminder from James 1 that you can find joy in even the darkest times. Even when you are going through trials and tribulations, you are strengthening your relationship with God. Count it all joy my friend. Another gem from the Bible in regards to joy is Proverbs 17:22 (NIV) "A cheerful heart is good medicine, but a crushed spirit dries up the bones." It even calls joy out as medicine! Your attitude—your joy—and outlook on life has a profound impact on your health; it says so in the Bible.

Spirituality in a faith-based wellness journey is your relationship with Jesus. Do you trust God? Do you truly believe? This goes beyond religion. This is your faith, your belief in Jesus Christ, your Savior who came to earth to free you from your sins. Do you spend time with Jesus? Romans 8:6 (NIV) says, "The mind governed by the flesh is death, but the mind governed by the Spirit is life and peace." The further away from your relationship with Jesus and your trust in God, the further away from peace, joy, and true health you get. In Romans, the death that's being referred to is not just a physical dying, but a separation from God. We are humans and we make mistakes—God knows this. You don't have to be perfect for God to love you. But when you are examining your spirituality, give yourself an honest assess- ment of how much you trust in God's plan for you. How often do you rely on "the flesh" or yourself to figure something out instead of giving it to God?

Recently, spirituality seems to be put on the back burner more and I don't think society sees it as an important piece of their health puzzle. Being a woman of faith, you already know what a profound impact your spirituality and belief in Jesus have on your life. And when you start to really align your life outside of church with your deeply held faith in God, you start to see your health improve. You begin to be in the right place at the right time, meet the right people who support and love you through your journey, and you feel your purpose. But even being a woman of faith, sometimes life takes you away from our faith. Sometimes you get in ruts when you haven't been to church or worship for a while or you haven't been praying as much, you took a break from reading the Bible, you don't feel close to God; you strayed in some way. And you'll find that oftentimes, once you pick your Bible back up, reach out to God, make Jesus your first thought and last thought of the day, your overall health begins to realign and feel better.

When your spirituality is strong, it is easier to identify which areas of health are out of alignment because you are working with your strong faith and values. Is your career in alignment with your faith? Do your relationships reflect your relationship with Jesus? Are you able to find joy through the difficult times? It's stressful to show up daily to a piece of your life in which you are diametrically opposed and which isn't in alignment with your faith, beliefs, and values.

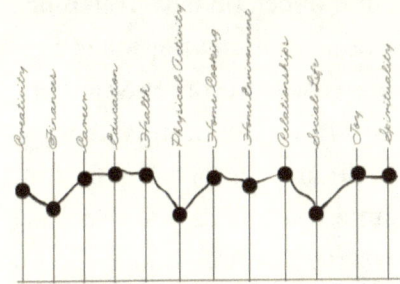

Example of Primary Foods Graph

A great tool you can use to assess how you feel you are doing in each of the primary foods is a simple line graph. Take a piece of paper and draw 12 vertical lines. On (or right next to) each of the lines, write one of the primary foods. Then you will make a dot on the line for how satisfied you are in each primary food. The further to the top of the line you make your dot, the more satisfied you are and the closer to the bottom of the line you make your dot, the less satisfied you are. Once you have one dot on each of the 12 primary foods, you can connect the dots and see which areas you are less satisfied with and which ones you are more satisfied with.

This is a great tool to use if you are feeling stuck or like something in your life has to change. It's a visual representation of how satisfied you are with each primary food. These ways of nourishing your body are vastly underrated and overlooked by most health care providers.

In the example, you can see that there are three primary foods that this woman feels least satisfied with in her life: finances, physical activity, and social life. These are the primary foods she would focus on first when creating changes to her lifestyle. She would make goals to create small changes and see if her satisfaction improves. This is not just a tool to use once and never reference again. It is something that can be done multiple times, perhaps quarterly or annually, to show progress as you work through primary foods you're not satisfied with. It is rare for anyone to be satisfied completely with every single area of primary food in their lives. This is not a way to shame yourself or make you feel like a failure. This is only meant to serve as a tool to support you in managing stress and improving health outcomes. When we start to focus on one primary food, it is common for another to then become less satisfying. That's okay! You are a human. You are doing an exceptionally amazing job. Keep going.

If you are looking at your graph from the primary foods tool or any of the considerations in this book and are freaking out because you think you have a lot of work to do; I want you to take a deep breath right now. If you are feeling overwhelmed that you need to change; I want you to take a deep breath right now. If you are looking at these intentional considerations and feeling good about the choices you make, I want you to take a deep breath anyway because breathing is awesome. Stress can be worse than the change sometimes. So please proceed with love and grace for yourself. You do not need to make a million changes all at once. Take small steps—one thing at a time.

Breathing

It sometimes feels silly to suggest someone breathe as a stress management tool because we are always breathing, right? Even if you held your breath and passed out, your body would automatically start breathing again. In Genesis 2:7 (NIV), you hear the story of how man became a living being: "Then the Lord God formed a man from the dust of the ground and breathed into his nostrils the breath of life…" We were created and made alive through God's breath. Breathing is such a foundational aspect of life—it *is* life. It's the difference between living and not living. And although it is an automatic function, your body's breathing cadences change due to many factors such as situations, weight, allergies, health issues, and environment.

When your body is experiencing stress, it activates something called your sympathetic nervous system which triggers your body's fight-or-flight response. Your breathing can become faster because your body demands more oxygen to prepare for action, creating rapid, shallow breaths. Because you start to breathe more shallow breaths, you start breathing from your upper chest instead of full, deep belly breaths, which can make you feel more breathless. Your breathing can become irregular, sometimes causing you to hold your breath or gasp more and it can also lead to hyperventilation. In cases of extreme stress, excessive breathing can lower carbon dioxide levels leading to dizziness, lightheadedness, or tingling sensations. Stress can also cause tightness in the chest muscles, making it feel harder to take deep breaths.

The way you breathe sends signals to your body through your nervous system. Short and shallow breathing feeds your sympathetic nervous system which supports your body's ability to fight-or-flight in a true dangerous situation, and slow, deep breathing signals your parasympathetic nervous system which is the part of the nervous system that allows you to calm down—rest and digest. Here are three breathing techniques you can try when you notice your body is in a stressed out state or to just use it as a daily mindfulness practice. Read your Bible while practicing these for a little added bonus!

Belly/Diaphragmatic Breathing

Have you ever watched a baby lying on his/her back breathe? Babies are the perfect example of belly breathing or diaphragmatic breathing. As a baby breathes in, you see his/her belly rise and fall. Somewhere along the way as humans age, breathing changes. Why? There are many possible reasons for this. There's a societal expectation of a hard, flat belly which isn't conducive to belly breathing since it expands your belly. People in general are more stressed out which tightens muscles and changes breathing patterns. Whatever the reason, you can practice belly breathing intentionally. Here's how:

-Sit or lie down on your back, whichever feels most comfortable to you

-Place one hand on your belly
-When you inhale, imagine a balloon in your belly and fill it with your breath
-Let your belly fall as you exhale
-Inhale and exhale for 4 counts each
-Continue until you feel relaxed

Finger-tracing Breathing

You will use both of your hands for this technique. Hold one hand up in front of your face and spread your fingers out. With the other hand, use your pointer finger to trace. Start with your pointer finger by your wrist (it doesn't matter if it's the left or right side of your hand, just at the base of your hand where it meets your wrist). As you trace up your finger, inhale and take a pause at the top. As you trace down your finger, exhale and take a pause at the bottom. When you have traced all of your fingers with your breathing and reached the other side of your wrist, you can trace your hand going the other direction. Do this for as long as you need to feel a sense of peace and calm with your breathing.

Alternate Nostril Breathing

When you are doing this breathing technique, you're going to breathe in one nostril and out the other while closing one nostril with a finger. Here's how it works:
-Place your thumb on one nostril and your ring finger on the other (don't plug them yet)
-Plug the nostril with the ring finger and inhale fully
-Hold for a moment while you switch which nostril is closed by taking your ring finger off and plugging the other nostril with your thumb
-Exhale

-Inhale through the same nostril you just exhaled
-Switch to plug your nostril with your ring finger and exhale
-Inhale through the same nostril you just exhaled
-Switch nostrils and repeat this process until you feel relaxed

Re-writing Your Narrative

Another tool for processing stressful events and roots to your emotions is to write out your story; write out the parts where you have felt the most stress. Once you have written out your story, take a step back and think about who you are today and how you have changed since the event. Then edit your story from a place of empowerment. You won't change what happened to you, but you will rewrite it from the woman you are today because of that event.

If you are still feeling very connected to who you were when the stressful event occurred, you can start in prayer. Pray that the Lord breaks those chains that tie you to your past so you can be free and you can work from a place of empowerment. If you are in a place where you have disconnected from the event enough where you have grown from the experience, but the emotions come back to you and impact your stress, this is a great strategy to process those last lingering emotions.

In the beginning of this book, I shared my story of my first period and I'm going to use this as my example since you are familiar with it. I'm also using this story because my emotional state around my first experience becoming a woman has impacted how I used to perceive my period for so many decades of my life. I am not who I was when I was a pre-teen, but the feelings of that day lingered. So here's how I would rewrite that story to show that scared girl all the love I feel for her now. I have underlined the parts I rewrote so you can see exactly how I did this.

The day I became a woman is a day I will never forget. My twelfth Christmas came the same way it always did—it was exciting and busy. I was blissfully unaware that one of my favorite holidays was about to change my life forever. When I went to the bathroom at my aunt's house, taking a much needed introvert break from my large family gathering, I looked down and saw them—the red drops of womanhood.

At first I doubted what I saw. This couldn't possibly be my period; I was just seeing things. Then reality started to sink in and along with it came the panic. I'm not at home! I'm not prepared for this! What should I do? I wasn't able to yell across the family party to get my mom to help me. However, if everyone found out, I knew I'd get the support I needed because my family loves me. This wasn't how it was supposed to happen, but God's plan doesn't always make sense. I'd spent the last couple years eager to become a woman—at home in the comfort of my bathroom stocked with all the proper feminine hygiene products. I had this idea that my mom would bring me a warm water bottle or heating pad to put on my abdomen and we would relax on the couch watching girly movies while eating our favorite snacks. This was far from my perfect image of how this was all going to go down, but I did it! I became a woman and tackled my first challenge with a quiet celebration—just me writing a new exciting chapter in my life.

Deep in the dark shadows of my brain hid the information I learned in fourth grade during "the talk," but we never covered what to do if you weren't in the comfort of your own home in any of the segments. I calmed myself down, stuffed some toilet paper in my underwear and silently revelled in my womanhood the rest of the evening.

After the excitement of Christmas quelled, the one friend I told in secret about my plunge into womanhood let the cat out of the bag to other people at school. At first, I wanted to crawl into a hole and never come out.

(Exaggeration was my love language at the time.) <u>But then I realized that</u> <u>because I was one of the very first girls in my friend group to get her period,</u> <u>others were excited for me and perhaps a little envious that they hadn't had</u> <u>theirs yet. What an honor it was to be the trailblazer for others; the experi-</u> <u>enced one who could support my friends as they became women themselves.</u>

I invite you to take some time to think about a pivotal time (or times) in your life that created a narrative that formed the way you see yourself or a situation when you wish someone loving could have supported you through. Think about your story: Where were you? What did you do? How did you feel—physically and emotionally? And if there's any negativity in your story, write it out and think about how you can transform that message into an empowered, loving, faith filled one. Imagine what kind of a woman you needed and what words you needed to hear at the time, and write the story from the perspective of her. This has the potential to release so many emotions, so do this with some tissues on hand. Even knowing the impact this technique has, when I rewrote my story above, I was shocked at how much emotion was released. You do not need to be a professional author to rewrite your narrative. You are already the woman the younger version of you needed.

As a mom myself, I can only hope that one day my own daughter has a positive experience around her period, free from shame or embarrassment and full of love and faith. When I share my story of my first period, this is the story I will share. What happened is what happened, but how I tell my story now is from a place of love. I tell it because I am now the woman who that little girl needed in that moment and perhaps the woman other women need, too.

Moving Forward in Faith

Feeling overwhelmed? You just read years' worth of information, so it's okay to feel like you need a minute to digest it all. Although this book is not meant to be a step-by-step guide, I don't want you to leave feeling so overloaded with information that you end up in, what I like to call, "analysis paralysis" and do nothing with what you just read. When it comes to overall health, here's what I suggest you keep the main focus: your faith.

Get close to Jesus. Create an everlasting relationship with Him and the rest will come. Without this foundation you will always be seeking; always be searching for the next best thing to make you feel good. You can eat a meticulously planned diet and be completely synced to your cycle, but without a meaningful relationship with God, there will always be something missing, creating gaps in your life as a Christian woman.

While keeping God the focus of your life, get in tune with your body. In a culture obsessed with quick fixes, I invite you to simply observe your body. Get a good feel for how your body functions and reacts before rushing to change anything.

When and if you do decide to make changes to your lifestyle and habits, be firm in your reason why. Do it because you want to live in alignment with God. Do it for the glory of God. Weight loss, energy levels, body image, etc. are all just added bonuses when you live for the glory of God. Make your body obedient because God wants it to be. Hold your thoughts captive because God commands you to. It's easy for your body to crave the pleasures of this world because your body doesn't care as much as your spirit cares about going to Heaven and being with Jesus.

Your body doesn't go with you. So it's your job to make your body obedient to the Holy Spirit.

Lifestyle change is best made when you make small, sustainable changes and go slowly. This work is not done quickly, but is the most impactful. One way some women are able to create these changes is by habit stacking. Habit stacking is taking what you already do and either modifying it or doing more at the same time. For example: I wanted to add an armpit detox with bentonite to my morning routine, so I put it on while I dry brushed my body which was already a part of my routine. It's finding a way to do more at the same time, which as a huge generalization, is something women typically excel at doing.

A word of caution for habit stacking, though: don't overdo it. Multi-tasking can be great, but it's really easy to slip into a life of constant distraction; always looking for ways to fit more into your day. I often hear women sharing that they wish they could find a way to sleep and be productive at the same time. Remember: sleeping is productive! But also, our society at large has become too rushed and on the go. The real challenge is doing only one thing at a time. I challenge you to be intentional with your routine and try only doing one thing at a time before you start habit stacking. Slow yourself down so you can be fully present in your actions. When you slow your pace down and focus on one task at a time, you're less likely to be distracted from God and your true life purpose and peace.

It's a bit of a paradox; society is very go-go-go yet sedentary. The go-go-go is rarely movement dependent. It's a rushed lifestyle driving or using public transit from here to there, sitting at work, coming home to warm up a quick meal, watch TV, scroll apps, buy online, order online, connect online. The go-go-go you may be experiencing is not as physical as it is mental and it drains you in a different way.

Have you ever felt physically tired? Maybe you had a really intense workout or went on vacation and walked 500 miles. Your body was probably sore, but overall you probably felt good. That's because when you are physically active, your body releases endorphins increasing your feelings of contentment.

On the contrary, have you ever felt mentally tired? Even if you've been sitting all day, you probably still feel tired and just want to sit more to relax. You might have a headache or feel slightly dizzy. You might experience some feelings of stress or anxiety from overthinking. Mental work does not signal endorphins and other feel good hormones like physical work. Have you ever gotten advice to overthink something when you're stressed out? I haven't. Usually the advice is to breathe, go outside, go for a walk, shake, dance—MOVE your body.

You were never meant to live disconnected from God. You were never meant to carry shame for the way you were made. Your body, with all its rhythms and seasons, was designed with care, created in the image of God, and entrusted to you not as a burden. Take care of your body as though you were taking care of the sacred home that it is.

To have faith in God is to have faith in the body He gave you. To honor your cycle is to honor the wisdom He placed within you. To nourish yourself—through food, through rest, through movement, through prayer—is to worship with your whole being.

This is embodied faith.

It is not just belief in your mind; it is trust in your bones. It is faith that moves, that breathes, that flows. It is knowing that your cycle is not something to be controlled or suppressed, but something to be supported with love and intention. It is rejecting what harms your health and choosing instead what brings vitality. It is listening, deeply, to what your body is asking for and responding with care, just as God does for you.

Romans 15:4 (NIV) reminds us that "for everything that was written in the past was written to teach us, so that through the endurance taught in the scriptures and the encouragement they provide we might have hope." Remember that the Bible is your 'owner's manual' and that your body is mirrored throughout scripture. Everything written for you in the Bible was put there with intent to guide and teach you about all aspects of life including your menstruation and health. The purpose of these teachings is to equip you with the tools to endure difficulties and to find comfort and encouragement in the face of challenges, ultimately leading to a firm hope in God.

I invite you now, as you close this book, to step into a new relationship with your body, one rooted in faith, not fear. Let your faith be something you feel in your flesh, in your blood, in your breath. Let it guide the way you nourish yourself, the way you rest, the way you show up for yourself and for others.

Let your cycle be a rhythm of renewal. Let your body be a place of prayer. This is what it means to have faith through the feminine: to see God's grace and glory in your body's rhythms. In your hormones. In your blood. In your breath. Let your life be a testimony of the glory of God.

Heavenly Father,

Thank You for the journey through these pages, for the wisdom of Your Word, and for the light You shine upon the women of Scripture. You have created us in Your image, fearfully and wonderfully made, with bodies that reflect the rhythms of life You designed.

Lord, as we reflect on the beauty and purpose of our creation, may we embrace the sacredness of our design. Just as You walked with the women of the Bible; Sarah, Rachel, and Hannah in their longing, Mary in her calling, the woman healed by Your touch—walk with us in every season of our lives. Let us see ourselves through Your eyes: cherished, valued, and set apart for Your glory.

Help us to honor the cycles You wove into our very being, knowing that even in the shedding of blood, there is renewal, healing, and a foreshadowing of the redemption found in Christ. May we carry this understanding forward, teaching future generations to see Your hand in every part of our existence.

Lord, let this book not just be words on a page, but a call to deeper faith, a reminder of our worth, and an invitation to draw closer to You. May we live boldly, love deeply, and trust fully in Your perfect design.

In the name of Jesus, who makes all things new, we pray.
Amen.

About the Author

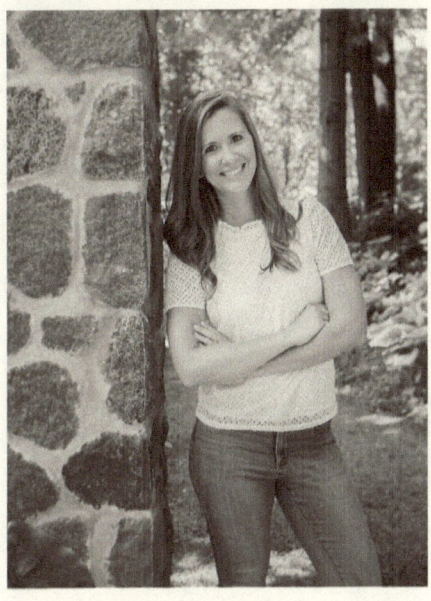

Alycia Hammer is a devoted wife, doting mother, Integrative Nutrition Health Coach specializing in women's hormones, and former public school educator. Based in her Wisconsin home, Alycia is passionate about helping women embrace God's design for their bodies through holistic, faith-based wellness. A God-fearing follower of Jesus, she weaves biblical truth into every aspect of her work, equipping women to steward their health with wisdom, grace, and purpose.

You can connect with Alycia via email at:
alycia.hammer@gmail.com
or through social media on Instagram @seventhwatchwomen
or Facebook Seventh Watch Women.

www.ingramcontent.com/pod-product-compliance
Lightning Source LLC
Chambersburg PA
CBHW031434120626
46545CB00006B/2394